Contents

Foreword

I have had many great blessings in my life but most have come only after great hurt and expense. Because of great marriage troubles and 10 kids worth of extreme family troubles plus some stray sheep we have taken in as well as financial woes and other major heartbreaks, I have often been driven to my knees to seek for guidance and comfort. Sometimes I get nowhere, but other times I have received both. As a result I have been able to understand and implement the principles that are in this book. These principles are not my own and to underscore that fact I include quotes from both ancient as well as modern prophets as well as dozens of other great men and women from all ages both ancient as well as modern. I have tried to give proper credit where credit was due.

I am a member in good standing of the Church of Jesus Christ of Latter-Day-Saints and , of course, I write from that point of view. I am married to my husband in a temple marriage where we were sealed for time and eternity and our children with us. What a great comfort that is in this world of turmoil and other uncertain beliefs. It seems that nearly everyone is crying out for this belief or that belief and the others are just crying. We all want happiness and are willing to do most anything to obtain it including lying, cheating, feeding our vanity or even doing drugs.

Our universe is based upon natural law. Even God Himself is bound to work within natural law. While gravity is just one of those natural laws it provides a very good example. It attracts everything. There are no exceptions. It is not capricious in its selection. Everything is attracted and to stay up you must obey the laws that allow it. The Wright brothers learned that when they figured out how to keep an airplane up in the air. A kite is doing that when it stays up in the air. Steve McQueen's character in the movie The Magnificent Seven, quoted a man that was falling from the top of a ten story building. As he passed every story he was heard to say "so far, so good". We assume that he was testing his theory that by exercising faith he could bypass, or overcome, or reverse that law of gravity. The movie never did explain the outcome of that poor man.

Our Heavenly Father has given us His Great Plan of Happiness. It also is based upon natural laws. Simply put; if we want to be happy we will follow those laws and as surely as day follows night we will become happy. And that is the whole purpose of this earth life. In fact there is no other way for us to become happy. The principles I outline in this book is a compilation of those natural law principles. This book is a primer. In other words I hope it is a base for you to begin your own study so that you too can be a part of God's Great Plan of Happiness.

Carry Your Own Sunshine

Copyright,   C Aug, 2019

The Author, Diana Sinclair, is a member of the Church of Jesus Christ of Latter-Day Saints and this book is written from that point of view. All of the opinions expressed by her in this book , however, are hers alone and in no way represent the official view of the Church.

Every effort has been made to give proper credit when quoting from another source however mistakes may be present and if so we apologize. Our goal is to always properly give credit where credit is due.

To contact the author or to purchase more copies of this book or other products in our store please go to www.unclesamsays.us or email ronsinclair2012@gmail.com

Chapter 1

Happiness

Why write a book titled *CARRY YOUR OWN SUNSHINE?*

Have you ever met someone who seemed truly happy? They were bubbling with enthusiasm. They were so full of the love of life, enjoying every minute. Did they have any problems? Not that you knew of. Were they rich, had servants to do their every bidding. Did they own nice things, a beautiful home, lushly landscaped, the newest vehicle and perhaps a plane or two. Did they travel all over the world on their own private jet, and vacation in the most scenic places on earth. Was everything perfect in their life, happily married with perfect children. Were they perfect in body and form. Did they have everything handed to them on a platter?

Some famous people who's parents were rich, like Paris Hilton, are looking for happiness. They are so worldly beautiful. A perfect size 2 or maybe 4, hair always in place, being seen at some of the most prestigious places, and having the news reporters and camera men follow them so closely they can barely even breath. Are they HAPPY? What is this elusive power that many people desire, to be happy. Some think it is wealth? Like looking for hidden treasures as in the gold rush in 1840's. When gold was discovered in Alaska, how many people perished traveling over the snow covered passes.

Carry your own sunshine. In the Bible in Matthew chapter 5:16 the Savior explains --

"Let your light so shine before men, that they may see your good works, and glorify your Father which is in heaven." The sunshine we carry is the Savior's and Heavenly Father's light. This is what brings true happiness, lasting enduring inner peace. This is a learning process, we can learn the correct principles for happiness. We have the greatest teacher in the world, Jesus Christ. It is because he understands us. He has been there and done that.

When the morning stars sang together, and ALL THE SONS OF GOD SHOUTED FOR JOY? Job 38:7. We actually shouted for JOY!!!! What has happened between then and now? Where is the joy, where is the happiness? How could we possibly be happy and joyful in the pre-existence knowing we were to come to earth and be tried and tested. Here we would experience pain and suffering, of all kinds, physical, mental and emotional. Here we would leave our beautiful heavenly home to come to an earth that is fallen, and where Satan rules.

Richard C. Edgley said, "An understanding of Christ's plan of redemption helps put (personal suffering) into perspective. In our preexistent state our Father in Heaven presented His plan for mortality, which Alma described as the 'plan of happiness' (Alma 42:8.) I believe we all understood that by coming to earth, we would be exposed to all of the experiences of earth life, including the not-so-pleasant trials of pain, suffering, hopelessness, sin, and death. There would be opposition and adversity. And if that was all we knew about the plan, I doubt if any of us would have embraced it, rejoicing, 'That's what I have always wanted-- pain, suffering, hopelessness, sin, and death.' But it all came into focus, and it became acceptable, even desirable, when an Elder Brother stepped forward and offered to go down and make it all right. Out of pain and suffering he would bring peace. Out of hopelessness He would bring hope. Out of transgression He would bring repentance and forgiveness. Out of death He would bring the resurrection of lives. And with that explanation and most generous offer, each, and every one of us concluded, 'I can do that. That is a risk worth taking.' And so we chose." Richard C. Edgley, "For Thy Good, " *Ensign*, May 2002, pg. 65)

Our memory has faded, there has been a veil placed over our minds, so we could be tried and tested, so the deep desires or our heart would be what motivated us in our thoughts and actions. OUR HEART THINKING WOULD BE WHAT WE REALLY DESIRED, AND THAT WOULD BE WHERE WE PLACED OUR ENERGY.

Neal A. Maxwell said,
        "We define the veil as the border between mortality and eternity; it is also a film of forgetting which covers the memories of an earlier experience. . . . . Without the veil, we would lose that precious insulation which would constantly interfere with our mortal probation and maturation. . . . . . Without the veil, we could not experience the gospel of work and sweat of our brow. . . . We are cocooned, as it were in order that we might truly choose. Once long ago, we chose to come to this very setting where we could choose. . . . . And the veil is the guarantor that our ancient choice will be honored." Neal A. Maxwell, BYU Speeches of the Year-1979 pages 219-220.

In 2nd Nephi 2:25, it says Adam fell that men might be; and men are, that they might have joy. Where is this joy, this happiness? Also in Moses 5:10. . . my eyes are opened, and in this life I shall have joy .

Wait a minute Lord, This earth life is so hard and so difficult, there is so much PAIN. I want to change my vote, well, maybe not change it but at least my shout for JOY. I think I would change it to a spoken tone, or perhaps even a whisper.

Neal A. Maxwell, has a very unique way of explaining the situation;

        "In some ways, our second estate, in relationship to our first estate, is like agreeing in advance to surgery. Then the anesthetic of forgetfulness settles in upon us. (One does) not de-anesthetize a patient to ask him again if the surgery should be continued . . . . Neal A. Maxwell, *BYU speeches of the Year*--1978, pages 151-152

But did we understand some of the things we would be asked to go through?

"When the time arrived for us to be advanced in the scale of our existence and pass through this mundane probation, councils were held and the spirit children were instructed in matters pertaining to conditions in mortal life, and reasons for such an existence. Joseph F. Smith, *Journal of Discourses*, 1:57

We were instructed, taught and trained and for further progression, to become like Heavenly Father, we needed to experience the good, and the evil and the consequences of both, even the Savior. I don't think He knew just how hard it would be.

Our Savior who created not only this earth, but ----"worlds without number have I created-"--Moses 1:33. In D.& C. 38:1,2 "Thus saith the Lord your God, even Jesus Christ, the Great I Am, Alpha and Omega, the beginning and the end, the same which looked upon the wide expanse of eternity, and all the seraphic hosts of heaven, before the world was made;

2. The same which knoweth all things, for all things are present before mine eyes---- "

The great God, Jehovah, who knew all things, yet when he was in the Garden of Gethsemane the pain was so intense, so much greater than he had imagined. In a revelation given through Joseph Smith, D.& C. 19:17,18----

17. But if they would not repent they must suffer even as I;

18. Which suffering caused myself, even god, the greatest of all, to tremble because of pain, and to bleed at every pore, and to suffer both body and spirit------and would that I might not drink the bitter cup, and shrink------"

Because of the intense pain, not only physically, but also spiritually, Jesus asked to be released.

"Then saith he unto them, My soul is exceeding sorrowful, even unto death: --------and he went a little further, and fell on his face, and prayed, saying, O MY FATHER IF IT BE POSSIBLE, LET THIS CUP PASS FROM ME:" Then the greatest words ever spoken--"NEVERTHELESS NOT AS I WILL, BUT AS THOU WILT." Matthew 26:38-39

Has the trials and burdens and heartaches of this life ever been so difficult to bare , so hard to endure, that you have prayed, Father, please just take me home. I don't want to be here any longer, I just want to be encircled about by your loving arms. I don't want to go on. Yet go on we must!! We can't quit. We won't drop out of the race. We were valiant in the pre-existence and we will be valiant here. How does the pre-existence relate to our happiness here on earth? Since we lived much longer there than here, there must be some tie that connects.

Spencer W. Kimball, *Teachings of Spencer W. Kimball* Page 30. Spencer W. Kimball said:

"And one day a great conference was held. .. . . there were billions of spirits attending. And he who presided at this meeting said to all of us who were assembled. . . . We will organize (an earth) and we will make it (special) for those souls to enjoy. . . . and we will let each one of you go down to the earth in your turn, and we will see if you will do all things that we command you. I WANT YOU TO BE HAPPY, AND ALL I ASK IS THAT .... YOU WILL DO CERTAIN THINGS THAT I SPECIFY. . . . . . . .every law I give you shall be for your good entirely."

What is the greatest desire of a parent? They want their children to be happy. They provide for them, care for them, teach and train them. They guide and direct them. The parents in watching a young child learning how to walk knows that in the learning process this child will fall down, and perhaps even get hurt. Does the parent then carry the child and never let it learn from it's own experiences how to balance, how to use the muscles, how to take the first faltering step?

Does the parent stop the learning process because the child may fall down and get hurt and cry? Of course not because they know the child will ultimately have more joy and happiness. The learning process is hard, but in the learning process muscles are developed, the child learns to walk on its own, and not only walk, but eventually it can have even much more freedom of movement, and run. The frustration and tears of the learning process are replaced by, new freedoms, and a happiness in being able to walk and run.

In the pre-existence we desired to become like Heavenly Father He had a physical body, we did not. He was perfect, we were striving for this. He explained how we could progress further by coming to earth, gaining a body and learning from our own experience, the good from the evil.

He explained that He would not leave us alone or without direction, but that He would provide a road map, He would show the way, by giving us commandments which, if we followed would lead the way back to Him and ultimate HAPPINESS & JOY. We could not experience a fullness of JOY without a physical body.

" the spirit and the body to be united never again to be divided, that they might receive a FULNESS OF JOY." D. & C. 138:17

"And we will prove them herewith, to see if they will do all things

12

whatsoever the Lord their God shall command them;

"And they who keep their first estate shall be added upon; and they who keep not their first estate shall not have glory in the same kingdom with those who keep their first estate; and they who keep their second estate shall have glory added upon their heads for ever and ever." Abraham 3:25-26

Heavenly Fathers's plan - - - is the PLAN OF HAPPINESS. Heavenly Father gave us agency, the right to choose.

". . . . . I prepared all things, and have given unto the children of men to be agents unto themselves." D.& C. 104:17

If there was not more than one choice how could we use our agency. It would be like taking a college exam. The test is supposed to be multiple choice, yet as we read through the questions we find there is only one choice for each answer. We can not choose. In heaven before we came to earth Satan said he could save all of Heavenly Father's Children. It was not a multiple choice test. It was fixed, according to Satan no one would fail. There was only one answer, you would be forced.

Joseph Smith said,
"The contention in heaven was-----Jesus said there would be certain souls that would not be saved; and the devil said he could save them all, and laid his (proposals) before the grand council, who gave their vote in favor of Jesus Christ. So the devil rose up in rebellion against God, and was cast down , with all those who put up their heads for him." (Joseph Smith, TPJS, page 357)

"It is not likely that the final decision of the contending armies took place immediately. Many, no doubt, were unsettled in their views, unstable in their minds, and undecided as to which force to join . . . . . and there may have been a long period before the division line was so strictly

13

drawn as to become unalterable . . . .. Among the two thirds who remained, it is highly probable that there were many who were not valiant in the war, but whose sins were of such a nature that they could be forgiven through faith in the future sufferings of the Only Begotten of the Father, and through their sincere repentance and reformation." (Orson Pratt, The Seer, Volume 1 Number 4, pages 54-54)

Through the scriptures and prophets we know that Satan rebelled , and one third of the host of heaven followed Lucifer. The rest of us followed the Savior, some more valiant than others, yet all who did not follow Satan will be able to come to earth and gain a physical body. Here each of us will be tried and tested to see if we will do all things the Lord commands us. Then according to our faithfulness here in this life with the veil placed over our minds, we will eventually receive our hearts desire. This test is designed so that what we really want we will get. The choice is ours.

In 2 Nephi 2:27 Wherefore, men are free according to the flesh; and all things are given them which are expedient unto man. And they are FREE TO CHOOSE LIBERTY AND ETERNAL LIFE, THROUGH THE GREAT MEDIATOR OF ALL MEN, or to choose captivity and death according to the captivity and power of the devil; FOR HE SEEKETH THAT ALL MEN MIGHT BE MISERABLE LIKE UNTO HIMSELF.

We are now here on earth, with a physical body. The test is real, there are many choices we can make. It is definitely multiple choice. We are free to choose, but the consequences are very real. How can we possible make the correct choices? Lehi in speaking to his sons explains how to choose and who to follow.

"And now, my sons, I would that ye should look to the great Mediator, and hearken unto his great commandments; and be faithful unto his words, and CHOOSE ETERNAL LIFE, according to the will of HIS HOLY SPIRIT; 2 Nephi 2:28 & 29

14

And not choose eternal death, according to the WILL OF THE FLESH AND THE EVIL WHICH IS THEREIN, WHICH GIVETH THE SPIRIT OF THE DEVIL POWER TO CAPTIVATE, TO BRING YOU DOWN TO HELL, THAT HE MAY REIGN OVER YOU IN HIS OWN KINGDOM.

Satan has pulled out all of the stops, he is raging a war against women. I don't think there is a woman in the United States, whether in the church or not, that is not concerned about their body. If they are not a perfect size 2 or 10, or whatever they think is ideal size, they are trying some sort of weight loss program, or have just finished one. The media is ever present with " these beautiful bodies." The trim, fit gorgeous drop dead girls and women.

Even going to the grocery store it is impossible to even pay for your food without seeing skinny beautiful women looking at you from the magazines that are always next to the checkout. Their hair is done with style, their clothes although very nice, nearly always very revealing, showing off their trim waist line, Their makeup is done with finesse even though they may be 65 they look 40. And if they are 40 they look 20. Now even the tweens, before becoming teenagers use make up and wear clothing that makes them look like pop stars.

Satan has put out his version of the perfect girl or woman., and the world is consumed with it. Anorexia, bulimia,. Is a way girls and even women, try to be the perfect size, it is more common than we realize. Satan has convinced the American woman that we will be extremely happy or the most happy if we lose 10 - 20 - or whatever. To be happy we must have the perfect size.

Movies, T.V. Videos, DVD's , all portray the wrong picture of woman. The packaging, the outside, the wrapping paper, It may be all glitter and glamor, but what is that person really like. What are the values.

15

What do they stand for. Are they an example of truth and righteousness.

I don't think St. Peter is going to say or put us into categorizes "O.K, You ladies that are a size twenty or more, the ones that are very hefty, you go over to these lower levels. You are just too round and flabby. Next, those of you who are too skinny, you know who I mean, you look like death warmed over, you get a little higher because there is not so much of you. Next , all the gorgeous, trim, beautiful, women, you get the highest most wonderful place of all."

That is ridiculous. I see woman of all shapes and sizes that are absolutely beautiful. An elderly , petite lady, maybe in her eighties, and in a wheel chair. She had health problems, she looked very fragile as if with the slightest gentle touch she might break - - - like a china doll. She was thin and tiny, but she has an enthusiasm and energy for life. I didn't know her, but I saw her in the temple. She was so happy. Her countenance was bright, and she radiated light and truth. To me it seemed as if she was ready to just step into the Celestial Kingdom. Did she fit any of the world's images of beauty. NO, she was elderly and had wrinkles, was confined to a wheel chair. but she definitely fits God's image of beauty. She had light and truth from within. She was beautiful.

Carol Dunkin was Stake Relief Society President. A kind warm caring lady. She talked in Stake Conference. In order to go to the stand she had a friend by her side, an oxygen tank. As she spoke you could hear the click - whoosh as the air moved through the tube, to keep her alive. She had a terminal disease that made breathing very difficult. Because of the medications she was on, her size had ballooned and her face was puffy and bloated. She had every reason to stay home and be miserable and feel sorry for herself. Her health was not going to get better, and she would never wear the size 8 or 10 or even 12's again. She knew she was going to die, YET, She had such enthusiasm, and in her face you could see the joy she had for life. Her inner beauty showed through her health challenges. She worked at the family history center and talked about the people that

16

came in, and how they helped them, and how she shared the gospel with non members who came in to work on their genealogy- - How enjoyable it was to help others learn about their ancestors. Never once did she mention her lack of health, but as she talked the whoosh - - click - - - whoosh - - - click seemed to dissolve into the background and we didn't even notice it.

How can we meet the world's standard of beauty? We don't have to, we can create our own and be an example to the world.

Wilford Woodruff said,

"There are two powers on the earth and in the midst of the inhabitants of the earth---the power of God and the power of the devil. In our history we have had some very peculiar experiences. When God has had a people on the earth, it matters not in what age, Lucifer, the son of the morning, and the millions of fallen spirits that were cast out of heaven have warred against God, against Christ, against the work of God, and against the people of God. And they are not backward in doing it in our day and generation. Whenever the Lord set His hand to perform any work, those powers labored to overthrow it." Wilford Woodruff, *Deseret Evening News*, 17 Oct. 1896)

In the pre-existence, our loving Heavenly Father was there teaching, guiding and directing us. He watched us and knew of our faithfulness, our talents and abilities, and potential. He knew who He could trust to move His work forward, especially in this great winding up scene, when Satan's powers are in full force. The Lord in His for-knowledge reserved some of his most valiant spirits for these latter days.

"Now the Lord had shown unto me, Abraham, the intelligences that were organized before the world was; and among all these there were many of the noble and great ones; "And God saw these souls that they were good, and he stood in the midst of them, and he said: These I will make my rulers; for he stood among those that were spirits, and he saw that they were good; and he said unto me :Abraham, thou art one of them;

17

thou wast chosen before thou wast born." Abraham 3: 22&23

John A. Widstoe said,

"In our pre-existent state, in the day of the great council, we made
a certain agreement with the Almighty. (God) proposed a plan, conceived
by Him. We accepted it. Since the plan is intended for all men, we became
parties to the salvation of every person under that plan. We agreed, right
then and there, to be not only saviors to ourselves, but measurably, saviors
for the whole human family. We went into partnership with the Lord. The
working out of the plan became then not merely the Father's work, and the
Savior's work, but also our work. The least of us, the humblest, is in
partnership with the Almighty in achieving the purpose of the eternal plan
of salvation. That places us in a very responsible attitude towards the
human race. By that doctrine, with the Lord at the head, we become
saviors on Mount Zion, all committed to offering salvation to the untold
numbers of spirits." John A. Widstoe, *Utah Genealogical & Historical
Magazine,* Oct. 1934, page 1890

Joseph Smith said,
"Every man who has a calling to minister to the inhabitants of the
world was ordained to that very purpose in the Grand Council of heaven
before this world was." (Joseph Smith, TPJS, page 365)

The war that began in the pre-existence continues, it is a battle for
the souls of men. Who will we choose to follow, The Savior, and the Great
Plan of Happiness, or Satan, and become miserable like unto him.
"Wherefore, men are free according to the flesh; and all things are given
them which are expedient unto man. And they are free to choose liberty
and eternal life, through the great Mediator of all men, or to choose
captivity and death, according to the captivity and power of the devil; for
he seeketh that all men might be miserable like unto himself." 2 Nephi
2:27

Gordon B. Hinckley stated:

"In this work there must be commitment. There must be devotion. We're engaged in a great eternal struggle that concerns the very souls of the sons and daughters of God. We are not losing. We are winning. We will continue to win if we will be true and faithful. We can do it. We must do it. We will do it. . . . . . .The war goes on. It is waged across the world over the issues of agency and compulsion. It is waged in our own lives, day in and day out, in our homes, in our work . . . ., it is waged over questions of love and respect, of loyalty and fidelity, of obedience and integrity . . . . We are winning and the future never looked brighter." Gordon B. Hinckley, *Ensign*, November 1986, Pages 44-45

Happiness is a choice, but as in all things there are correct principles to follow in order to reach the desired results. I have taught music lessons for years. It is always interesting to work with a new student. Their attitude, abilities, talent, and interests vary. Some have taken lessons before from another teacher and if that instructor was positive, and kind it affected the person for good. However if the teacher was very critical, little if any praise, some students were afraid, and shy, and not willing to try for fear of being criticized.

Some teens and adults had the idea that if they had several lessons they would be able to play beautifully in a couple of weeks. I would gently try and explain, learning an instrument is like learning a foreign language. It takes time and a lot of practice.

"There is a law, irrevocably decreed in heaven before the foundations of this world, upon which all blessings are predicated-- And when we obtain any blessing from God, it is by obedience to that law upon which it is predicated." D. & C. 103:20-21.

God wants us to be happy and to feel his great love for us, 1 Nephi

19

11:22,23 Love of God is joyous to the soul. Happiness is the result of correct choices, obedience to God's commandments brings true lasting happiness. Happiness is the result of our thinking, our attitude, "As a man thinketh so is he" This is one of the things we are to learn. The gospel plan is "The Plan of Happiness"

The Beatitudes in Matthew 5, are a blue print. It starts with what we think about. Bad things happen to us all, even the Savior was not spared, yet he did not dwell of the terrible injustices for to him, He was perfect, and deserved no wrong done to him, Yet during his earthly ministry, no matter, what was said about him, even calling him Belezubub (meaning the Devil), criticizing him at every turn, calling his good works evil because it was done on the Sabbath. The Pharisies striving to find any fault , in his good deeds, so they could kill him.

JESUS WENT ABOUT DOING GOOD.

Moroni is a very good example of learning to be Happy. He is the sole survivor of the Nephites, the rest dissenting, going over the Lamanites, or being hunted down and killed. He is focusing on the joy that will come, the peace and happiness is talking about the redemption of man, when we are brought back into the presence of the Lord, being resurrected. "And then cometh the judgment of the holy One upon them; and then cometh the time that he that is filthy shall be filthy still; and he that is righteous shall be righteous still; **he that is HAPPY SHALL BE HAPPY STILL;** and he that is unhappy shall be unhappy still. Mormon 9:14

Being happy is a learning process, following correct principles.

Church News, 24th November 2001;

Marjorie P. Hinckley celebrates 90th birthday. Asked what she considers a good birthday present, she said, "JUST TO BE ALIVE, TO BE

20

ABLE TO PUT MY SHOES ON AND GO." Sister Hinckley claims no particular formula for living a long and happy life, beyond being optimistic. "IF YOU'RE NOT OPTIMISTIC, LIFE IS REALLY A BURDEN," she observed.
"YOU OUGHT TO LOOK FOR THE SUNNYSIDE." As for challenges, she has a simple philosophy: "YOU JUST HAVE TO FACE UP TO EVERY DAY AND NOT BE AFRAID, BUT KNOW THAT LIFE IS GOOD AND THAT THINGS WILL WORK OUT."

Whenever darkness fills our minds, we may know that we are not possessed of the Spirit of God, and we must get rid of it. WHEN WE ARE FILLED WITH THE SPIRIT OF GOD, WE ARE FILLED WITH JOY, WITH PEACE AND WITH HAPPINESS NO MATTER WHAT OUR CIRCUMSTANCES MAY BE; FOR IT IS A SPIRIT OF CHEERFULNESS AND OF HAPPINESS." Gospel Truth, 1:19-20
From *D.& C. Student Manuel*---pg 161

This earth life is the test, we are like Lehi as he explained his dream. He was in a dark and dreary wilderness. It was very confusing, he didn't know where to go or how to get out of the situation. Then he saw a man in a white robe, who motioned for Lehi to follow him.
By following this man, Lehi didn't suddenly leave this dark place, in fact he traveled for many hours in darkness. Then Lehi began to pray that the Lord would have mercy on him. He prayed - - prayer is available to all of us at any time, in any circumstance, in the darkest pit, in sadness, in sorrow, in grief or pain. When Abraham prayed he was on the alter ready to be sacrificed, - - - and the Lord came to him.

So with Lehi's fervent prayer he was brought out of the darkness in to the light, and there he saw a tree - - "**whose fruit was desirable to make one happy.**" Lehi explains the fruit, that it was exceedingly white, he had never seen anything this brilliant white before. As he partakes of the fruit, he is awed or wondered at how he felt.

Verse 12; And as I partook of the fruit there of it filled my soul with exceedingly great joy. 1 Nephi 11: 22 & 23, the angel is showing Nephi the dream his father had. V. 22 And I answered him saying: Yea, it is the love of God, which sheddeth itself abroad in the hearts of the children of men; wherefore, it is the most desirable above all things. V. 23 And he spake unto me, saying: Yea, and the most joyous to the soul.

GOD GAVE US A GREAT PATTERN TO FOLLOW IN CHOOSING TO BE HAPPY.

Each of us has many responsibilities, and work to do. Many times it can be overwhelming and very frustrating to tackle a big job, it is like they say, how do you eat an elephant,,,, one bite at a time.

There is the story of a man who had a large wood pile that was quite a walk from his house where he had a fireplace, each time he thought of the job of moving all of that wood he kept putting it off until another day. He figured it would take him forever. He was telling his neighbor who was visiting one day, and showed him the huge pile, and explaining what a long time it would take him. The wise neighbor saw that the wood was stacked near the out- house out door toilet, which of course was used during the day. The man said, each time you come out here to take a break, carry some wood back with you and stack it near your house.

The farmer decided to take his advice, he was pleasantly surprised that in less than a week had moved all the wood. It wasn't such a big job after all. Take any large task and divide it into sections. You will feel a great sense of accomplishment, when rather than taking weeks or months to complete a project, you can take joy and feel rewarded with each small section you complete. You CAN feel good about what you have done by taking bite sized bits, rather than trying to eat the whole elephant in one sitting.

Chapter 2

AGENCY

Harold B. Lee, in his book *Stand Ye in Holy Places*, p.235, said "Next to life itself, free agency is God's greatest gift to mankind, providing thereby the greatest opportunity for the children of God to advance in this second estate of mortality." What a marvelous gift Agency is, that is the only way we can progress, if we didn't have choices we wouldn't grow and learn. Everyday we have many choices to make. We are being enticed by Satan, he is counterfeit, he is the great deceiver, his whole purpose is to make us as miserable as himself. He will make black look white, and white look black.

Nephi explains this so well in 2 Nephi 2:26,27. Because Christ redeemed us from the fall, we have become free forever, knowing good from evil; to act for our selves and not to be acted upon. We have the freedom to choose, even when bad things happen to us, through no fault of our own, we can still choose our response.

Satan wants us to sin because that turns us away from God because the Spirit withdraws when we are sinning. Satan's false teaching are roaring in our ears, and if we don't listen carefully we may not be able to hear the quiet promptings of the Spirit.

As the Primary song says, "Through the Still Small Voice, the spirit speaks to me to guide me, to **SAVE** me from the evil I may see. If I try to do what's right, he will lead me thru the night, Direct me, protect me, and give my soul his light." (*Children's Songbook*, page 106 & 107) " The Still Small Voice"

Brittney Ann S. In the New Era, May 2011 pg. 46-47. Tells what happened to her at college. Her mother had taught her the gospel and was always reminding her "you Know what's Right". One evening her roommate invited her to a party. As her friend led her to the apartment Brittney was surprised that the door was locked, and the only way to get in was to identify who you were. Brittney didn't concern herself about it speculating that they probably didn't want a huge crowd of people at the party and this was a way to control how many were there. As she walked into the room she had an uneasy feeling come over her, but she just brushed it off thinking the reason she felt that way was because she didn't know the people. Later on she saw some of the college students going in and out of a door that led to the back of the apartment. She asked her roommate who had invited her and been to these parties before what was going on.

"That's where all the alcohol was and that they had to keep it back there in case the police showed up."

Brittney then realized that the uneasy feeling she had was the Holy Ghost telling her something was not right, that she should not be there. When Brittney told her roommate that she was going back to her own apartment, her friend did everything she could to get Brittney to stay. It was an emotional dilemma what to do. She didn't want to offend her friend, and she knew she didn't have to go into the back room, that way she would still be there but not participate in the drinking, yet if the police showed up they would not believe she was innocent. The words of her mom popped into her mind. "Brittney, you know what is right." She immediately left the party and went to her own apartment, she said, even though the police didn't show up, she was glad she followed the promptings of the Spirit, by remembering what her mother had taught her. "You know what is right."

25

Brittney used her agency to recognize the impressions of the Holy Ghost, reminding her of the valuable teachings of her mother, and then to have the courage to leave, or flee, as Joseph of Egypt from Potiphers wife.

My husband and I go on a weekly date, it gives us one on one time, in fact my husband calls it our "Marriage Insurance." Sometimes, a movie, or dinner, or picnic, or a drive up in the mountains Mount Charleston just a 40 minute drive from our home - to get cooled off from the Las Vegas heat, in the summer, or going in the winter to enjoy the snow. One evening we looked at the reviews of the movies and saw a fun comedy that was playing close by. It was rated P.G. 13, so we figured it would be a fun entertaining evening.

The first 10 or 15 minutes was enjoyable showing married couples and how they related to each other in a humorous way. Then the producers started adding light suggestive material, I got this uncomfortable feeling but I just put it in the back of my mind, thinking, the first part was good I'm sure it will go back to being a clean show. Yet the longer we stayed the more suggestive the movie became. I could not squish the uneasy feeling I had. The thought came to me, "Get up and leave, you can walk out of a movie" I mentioned this to my husband that we should walk out, yet we both still sat till the end. We were both feeling yucky and commented to each other what a bad show this was. Looking in hind sight we were both thinking we should have left the show after the first 15 minutes.

The next day Sunday morning before church I was pondering on what to do in the future. I was listening to the B. Y. U. Channel. They had an L. D. S. worship service on and the speaker was talking about Sodom & Gomorrah. How Lot first pitched his tent facing Sodom, & then later on he moved into the city. Of his family only his 2 daughters and wife left with the angel, then Lot's wife looked back. The speaker said it was not just looking back, she desired to go back and be there, her heart was there.

He explained we must keep the evil out. We must shun evil, like Joseph of Egypt, he ran from Potoipher's wife. He said if we don't - -- "We are like a man in front of a firing squad - - -
then we give them the bullets. This next sentence was aimed directly at me, "HAVE THE COURAGE TO WALK OUT OF A MOVIE" This hit me right between the eyes. How did he know about the movie we had watched last night and how uncomfortable we both felt. I know the Lord meant for me to hear his words. In my prayers that morning I asked Heavenly Father to forgive me, and I also said I would have the courage to walk out. I explained this to my husband and he readily agreed.

Several nights before this our neighbors Johnnie and Michelle's car was stolen. Michelle got home from work late in the evening, and as she was doing some chores noticed the trash needed emptying so grabbing the bag headed out side. Something was wrong! Her car was gone; she had parked it in the driveway just 30 minutes ago. It was close to midnight , about 11:30 P.M. "Where's My Car!: Johnnie immediately called the police and got in his car and decided to find it. He cruised the neighborhoods checking each car that went by. Finally he saw it. He knew it was his car because he recognized the head lights. He again called the cops, and started to chase them, but he had to do a U-Turn, so they got away, however a few blocks away he found the car with the doors flung open and beer in the back. It is a miracle he found it.

After we got home from our date we were up for another hour. Our neighbor, Johnnie called and said, "Your side window on your Yukon is down, or somebody might have broken into it. This was 11:00 P.M. Several months before the window behind the driver's seat would not stay up, so my husband put packaging tape to hold it up. Clear tape, but if you looked closely you could see it. All someone had to do was pull off the tape, then the window would fall down. Well that is what happened. They crawled inside and tried to get it started. The Yukon has a great security

27

system, but since no doors were opened it didn't go off. They tried to jimmy the ignition with a screw driver, but by then the alarm was sounding with the horn honking. That is when Michelle heard the alarm, and Johnny called us. We were so grateful they did not succeed in stealing it. Ron & I wondered if we had left the movie - Walked out - if this might not have happened.

President David O. McKay said, "God gave to man part of his dignity. He gave to man the power of choice, and no other creature in the world has it. So he placed upon the individual the obligation of conducting himself as an eternal being. You cannot have any greater gift that could come to man or woman than the freedom of choice. You alone are responsible, and by wielding and exercising that freedom of choice, you grow in character, you grow in intelligence, you approach divinity, and eventually you may achieve that high exaltation. This is a great obligation. Very few people appreciate it. The roads are clearly marked - - - one offering animal existence, the other life abundant. Yet, God's greatest creation - - man - - often is content to grovel on the animal plane."

The Prophet Joseph Smith taught:

"HAPPINESS IS THE OBJECT AND DESIGN OF OUR EXISTENCE; and will be the end thereof, if we pursue the path that leads to it; and this path is virtue, uprightness, faithfulness, holiness, and keeping all the commandments of God.

"IN OBEDIENCE THERE IS JOY AND PEACE. AND AS GOD HAS DESIGNED OUR HAPPINESS . . . . . , HE NEVER HAS----HE NEVER WILL . . . GIVE A COMMANDMENT TO HIS PEOPLE THAT IS NOT CALCULATED IN ITS NATURE TO PROMOTE THAT HAPPINESS WHICH HE HAS DESIGNED." (History of the Church, 5:134-135.)

If happiness is the object and design of our existence, then it stands to reason that we should be happy all of the time. If a person looks around them, and perhaps even in the mirror we usually don't see someone who is happy 24 hours a day, every day. There must be more answers.

President Faust stated:

"Happiness is not given to us in a package that we can just open up and consume. Nobody is ever happy 24 hours a day, seven days a week. Rather than thinking in terms of a day, we perhaps need to snatch happiness in little pieces, learning to recognize the elements of happiness and then treasure them while they last." Ensign, Oct 2000, an article by President James E. Faust entitled "Our Search for Happiness", page 2

Happiness is a choice, it is a decision, a conscious choice. It is directing our mind on what we decide to focus on. What we think about. We are not always able to choose what happens to us because God has given everyone of his children agency, and in using that agency many times we make wrong choices that affect not only ourselves, but many others through our incorrect decisions. If someone decides to drink and then to drive and then because he is drunk has an accident, innocent people may be hurt or even killed. The person who is hurt or killed, did not choose this. Where is agency in this?

God has given us the gift of agency, therefore because none of us are perfect, many wrong choices are made, and some have terrible consequences that follow, not only to the person who used his agency unwisely, but many times to innocent victims .

Richard L. Evans said,

"If God wants us to be happy, and he gave us the plan of happiness, how can we be happy? Especially since much of our heartache and pain is caused by the actions of others. This is where faith comes in, faith in

29

Heavenly Father and in His Son, Jesus Christ. God loves us so much that He wants us to have a fulness of joy. In His great love and wisdom He knows that if He carried us throughout this earth life and we never had any trials, or problems, or heartaches, that if every day was like being in the Garden of Eden we could not grow and develop and become like Him."

Neal A. Maxwell, stated,

"Quite understandably, the manner in which things unfold seem to us mortals to be so natural. Our not knowing what is to come (in the perfect way that God knows) thus preserves our agency completely. When, through a process we call inspiration and revelation, we are permitted to tap that divine data bank, we are accessing the knowledge of God."
(Neal A. Maxwell, *BYU Speeches of the Year 1978,* page 153)

The scripture from Proverbs 3:5 & 6 Explains how to have this faith in Heavenly Father. "Trust in the Lord with all thine heart; and lean not unto thine own understanding. In all thy ways acknowledge him and he shall direct thy paths."

He is directing our lives, He knows what we need to become like Him. There are so many unanswered questions in this life that we must have faith and trust Him. Especially in our own Gethsemane when the trials are so difficult we want to give up.
D.& C. 122:7 explains this well as the Lord is talking to Joseph Smith in his terrible afflictions. . . . . . . "if the very jaws of hell shall gape open the mouth wide after thee, know thou, my son, that all these things shall give thee experience, AND SHALL BE FOR THY GOOD."

The Lord explains another reason for agency;

"That every man may act in doctrine and principle pertaining to futurity, according to the moral agency which I have given unto him, that every man may be accountable for his own sins in the day of judgement."

30

D.& C. 101:78

God does not take away men's agency. That is given to us from Him. Many innocent people have been hurt or even killed because of the actions of others, yet the Lord suffers this to happen so that when the wicked are punished, God's judgements are just.

This is explained so well in the Book of Mormon. Alma and Amulek were forced to watch the terrible destruction of the women and children being killed by fire.

Amulek in his sorrow wants to save the women and children from this pain.

Alma 14: 10, 11, "And when Amulek saw the pains of the women and children who were consuming in the fire, he also was pained; and he said unto Alma; How can we witness this awful scene? Therefore let us stretch forth our hands, and exercise the power of God which is in us, and save them from the flames."

Alma must have also felt deep sorrow at this heart wrenching scene. Yet he was so close to the Spirit that he received this deeper insight. "But Alma said unto him: The Spirit constraineth me that I must not stretch forth mine hand; for behold the Lord receiveth them up unto himself, in glory; and he doth suffer that they may do this thing, or that the people may do this thing unto them, according to the hardness of their hearts, that the judgements which he shall exercise upon them in his wrath may be just; and the blood of the innocent shall stand as a witness against them, yea, and cry mightily against them at the last day."

In the Bible Dictionary, page 777 In defining the word suffer it says; " Suffer-- to permit, allow. Also used in its current meaning of enduring and tolerating pain, affliction, or an uncomfortable situation." Did God want this to happen? No!! Did he allow it to happen? Yes!

31

Why??? These were righteous women and children. They were received into the arms of God and would receive joy and happiness in being in His presence.

And the wicked?? Because God is both just and merciful, he allowed this to happen so that his judgements against them may be just. The Lord will heal those who have been so badly hurt, God will wipe away all tears from their eyes, while the wicked who have not repented will suffer till their debt is paid. "And God shall wipe away all tears from their eyes and there shall be no more death, neither sorrow, nor crying, neither shall there be any more pain; for the former things are passed away."

"He that overcometh shall inherit all things; and I will be his God, and he shall be my son." "But the fearful, and unbelieving, and the abominable, and murderers, and whoremongers, and sorcerers, and idolaters,, and all liars, shall have their part in the lake which burneth with fire and brimstone; which is the second death." Revelation 20:4, 7,8

We cannot always choose what happens to us, but we can choose our response. We can choose how we act or react to a situation. We decide what we think, therefor we choose our response. The Savior was the perfect example of this. He was accused, spit upon, reviled against. Isaiah explains:

"He is despised and rejected of men, a man of sorrows, and acquainted with grief: and we hid as it were our faces from him; he was despised, and we esteemed him not. Surely he hath borne our griefs, and carried our sorrows; yet we did esteem him stricken, smitten of God, and afflicted. But he was wounded for our transgressions, he was bruised for our iniquities; the chastisement of our peace was upon him; and with his stripes we are healed. " Isaiah 53: 3-5

Our Lord and Savior suffered, mental, emotional and physical abuse. He was reviled against, He was spit upon , He was mocked, a crown of thorns was placed on His head. He was whipped and then the worst death possible, He was crucified. Such pain we can not even imagine. During all of this agony He said, "Father, forgive them; for they know not what they do." Luke 23:34

Jesus not only taught us to forgive by His words, but He also showed by His example. He lived the life He wanted us to live. He said come follow me. He forgave, He showed us how.
During His darkest hours His thoughts were on others. " When Jesus therefore saw his mother, and the disciple standing by, whom he loved, he saith unto his mother, Woman, behold they son! Then saith he to the disciple, Behold thy mother! And from that hour that disciple took her unto his own home."   John 19: 26 & 27

How did the Lord respond? By love, kindness and forgiveness. He had every reason to be angry, to get vengeance, to get even, to retaliate. He did not. Jesus set the perfect example. How do we deal with the feelings we have? They are real. Everyone of us at times has been treated unkindly, or even untruths spoken about us. People may have gotten angry at you for no apparent reason, or perhaps there was a misunderstanding. You may have been emotionally, or physically abused. This life is real and injustices happen to all of us.

There are many examples in the scriptures, some of my favorites are in the Book of Mormon. I read about Nephi and I marvel at his great spiritual strength, and his unwavering faith. He saw visions, and angels. He was a prophet, and yet at times he struggled. In 2nd Nephi chapter 4 Nephi is writing about the great blessings God has given him.

In verses 20-25- - --My God hath been my support- - - - - -He hath filled me with his love- - - - He hath confounded mine enemies- - - - - Behold, he hath heard my cry by day, and he hath given me knowledge by visions in the nighttime. - - - - - - My voice have I sent up on high; and angels came down and ministered unto me. - - - - - And upon the wings of his Spirit hath my body been carried away upon exceedingly high mountains. And mine eyes have beheld great things- - - -Yet even Nephi with his great spiritual strength had so many trials and hardships that he struggled. In verse 27, he explains this great inner conflict.

"And why should I yield to sin, because of my flesh? Yea, why should I give way to temptations that the evil one have place in my heart to destroy my peace and afflict my soul? WHY AM I ANGRY BECAUSE OF MINE ENEMY?"

Nephi was ANGRY----- as we look at the circumstances surrounding Nephi, we can understand why he was angry. His father Lehi had just died and his older brothers Laman and Lemuel wanted to kill him. Not only then but they had tried before, and he and his wife and children, and Nephie's younger brothers Jacob and Joseph had suffered much because of Laman and Lemuel's actions.

Here is a key factor in learning to be happy. Recognize, or acknowledge our feelings. Nephi did this, he was angry. He didn't pretend this situation did not exist. It was very real and hurt deeply. He didn't bury the feelings or emotions

Nephi was angry, but he didn't stay there. He used great spiritual and mental energy to call on the Lord. He gave his burdens to the Lord. He cried with all of the energy of his soul for the Lord's help He realized that staying angry took away his PEACE. gain in verse 27 "Yea, why should I give way to temptations, THAT THE EVIL ONE HAVE PLACE IN MY HEART TO DESTROY- --- --- -MY PEACE- - - - - AND AFFLICT MY SOUL?"

Nephi recognized his feelings, and he pleaded mightily with the Lord to help him.. He told the Lord all of his feelings and asked for His help. Verse 31 & 33 "O Lord, wilt thou redeem my soul? Wilt thou deliver me out of the hands of mine enemies?---- wilt thou make away for mine escape before mine enemies!"

Nephi used his agency to change his focus. Verse 28 "AWAKE, MY SOUL! No longer droop in sin. REJOICE, O MY HEART, and give place no more for the enemy of my soul."Then Nephi turned his thoughts to the Lord, this was Nephi's desire. Verse 30 "REJOICE, O my heart, and cry unto the Lord, and say: O Lord, I will praise thee forever; yea, MY SOUL WILL REJOICE IN THEE, MY GOD, AND THE ROCK OF MY SALVATION."

Nephi put his complete faith and trust in the Lord. Verse 34 & 35 "O Lord, I have trusted in thee, and I will trust in thee forever.- - - - - -Yea, I know that God will give liberally to him that asketh. Yea, my God will give me, if I ask not amiss; therefore I will lift up my voice unto thee; yea, I will cry unto thee, my God, the rock of my righteousness. Behold, my voice shall forever ascend up unto thee, my rock and mine everlasting God."

Steve F. Gilliland gave examples of two ways we can react to Injustice. " Two negative reactions to injustice are common. One is to deny what is going on inside. We may say to ourselves: "What that person said hurts. - - - - - I shouldn't let it affect me. - - - - -It really doesn't bother me. - - - - I'm fine."

"Yet ignoring our feelings does not necessarily make them go away. They may continue to negatively influence our behavior in subtle ways without our even being aware of it"
Steve continues, "Another reaction is to wallow in our feelings, allowing them to become an obsession. We may talk about an individual who has wronged us to anyone who will listen. Even if we never seek revenge, we may continue to dream of doing so. An old sore is never permitted to heal when it is continually rubbed." by Steve F. Gilliland "Forgiveness -- Our Challenge and Our Blessing". *Ensign* August 2004 pg. 45 & 46.

35

In order for us to move forward on the road to happiness we must recognize our feelings, our hurts, angers, sorrows, fears. We pray mightily to the Lord and ask His help in moving past them , to change our focus. We put our complete faith and trust in the Lord knowing He is there directing our path, and that whatever happens is for our experience our learning and our good

Nephi, a great prophet cried mightily unto the Lord, because of his enemies. These enemies were not in a distant land , They were not just his neighbors across the street , they were not a distant relative. They were his very own brothers Laman and Lemuel.

Nephi cried mightily to the Lord, about his enemies , his borthers Laman and Lemuel.
"I Nephi, did cry much unto the Lord my God, because of the anger of my brethren." 2 Nephi 5:1

What happened?? God does not take away the agency of others, he allows them to choose. Nephi was a prophet, and prayed mightily to the Lord. Did God hear Nephi's prayers? Yes!! Did Lamen and Lemuel change   their attitude toward Nephi? NO! In fact they were even more angry with Nephi and more determined to kill him.

The Lord warned Nephi to flee in the wilderness.

"Wherefore, it came to pass that I, Nephi, did take my family, and also Zoram and his family, and Sam, mine elder brother and his family, and Jacob and Joseph, my younger brethren, and also my sisters, and all those who would go with me. And all those who would go with me were those who believed in the warnings and the revelations of God; wherefore, they did harken unto my words.

"And we did observe to keep the judgments, and the statutes and

36

the commandments of the Lord in all things according to the law of Moses. 2 Nephi 5: 5,6,10

Another example from the Book of Mormon is in Alma Chapter 31. Alma had received news that the Zoramites were perverting the ways of the Lord. They had fallen into great errors, for they would not observe to keep the commandments of God. Neither would they observe the performances of the church, to continue in prayer and supplication to God daily, that they might not enter into temptation.

The Zoramites had built synagogues where they did worship one day of the week. In the center of the synagogue they built a small tower which was high above the head. There was only room for one person to stand. When someone wanted to worship they would stand on the top of this tower and stretch forth their hands toward heaven, and cry with a loud voice

In verses 16, 17 & 18
"Holy God, we believe that thou hast separated us from our brethren, and we do not believe in the tradition of our brethren, which was handed down to them by the childishness of their fathers; but we believe that thou hast elected us to be thy holy children; and also thou hast made it known unto us that there shall be no Christ..

"But thou art the same yesterday, today, and forever; and thou hast elected us that we shall be saved, whilst all around us are elected to be cast by thy wrath down to hell; for the which holiness O God, we thank thee; and we also thank thee that thou hast elected us, that we may not be lead away after the foolish traditions of our brethren which doth bind them down to a belief of Christ, which doth lead their hearts to wander far from thee, our God.

"And again we thank thee, O God, that we are a chosen and a holy people. Amen."

Alma recognized his feelings as it says in these verses. Verse 1- - - - "-When Alma saw the iniquity of the people his heart again began to sicken. Verse 24- - - - As he saw this wickedness his heart was grieved. Verse 30 - - - - and such wickedness among this people doth pain my soul.. Verse 31 - - - O Lord, my heart is exceedingly sorrowful "- --

Alma didn't try and hide his feelings, he acknowledged them. He gave them all to the Lord. "Lord this is how I feel and this is why."

Then Alma asked the Lord to help him change his focus, his thinking.

"- WILT THOU COMFORT MY SOUL IN CHRIST. O Lord, wilt thou grant unto me that I may have strength, that I may suffer with patience these afflictions which shall come upon me, because of the iniquity of this people."Verse 31- - -

Alma asked the Lord for help, he asked specifically for what he desires.   Then he also includes in his prayers the brethren who were with him, Ammon, Aaron, Omner, Amulek , Zeezrom, and also his two sons.

Alma did not pray that the trial of seeing this great wickedness be taken away, because the Lord gives agency to all men. But he did pray that through this trial his soul and the hearts of his brethren would be comforted.

" O Lord, wilt thou comfort my soul, and give unto me success and also my fellow laborers who are with me - - - -even all these wilt thou comfort, O Lord. Yea, wilt thou COMFORT THEIR SOULS IN CHRIST."Verse 32

In verses 34 and 35 Alma asked for help in bringing the Zoramites to the Lord. He prays for success, power and wisdom in this great task.

"O lord, wilt thou grant unto us that we may have success in Bringing them again unto thee in Christ.

"Behold, O lord, their souls are precious, and many of them are our brethren; therefore, give unto us O Lord, Power and wisdom that we may bring these, our brethren, again unto thee."Verse 36
 as he clapped his hands upon them, they WERE FILLED WITH THE HOLY SPIRIT.

And the Lord provided for them - ---- and he also gave them strength, that they should suffer no manner of afflictions, save it were SWALLOWED UP IN THE JOY OF CHRIST." Verse 37

Alma's focus was on the Savior and helping others. Also his request was granted because of his prayer and great faith.

"Now this was according to the prayer of Alma; and this because HE PRAYED IN FAITH." Verse 38,

Our agency is God given, God wants us to be free to make choices, and then to be accountable for our choices. Satan wants it the other way around, to have us choose any action we want, because it makes us feel good. Then if there are problems resulting from the choice , we blame others for our actions. My parents, my wife, my boss, my job, etc. So when things go wrong it is never their fault. It is like in the Book of Mormon, when a wicked king rules.

In the book "How to Hug a Porcupine" by Dr. John Louis Lund in chapter 6 pages 87 & 88 explains "A difficult truth to accept is that no one can change toxic people. They can only change themselves. "Can toxic people change?" Is a different question. Yes, absolutely; but the desire to replace unhealthy behaviors with healthy ones has to be the decision of the toxic person."

The only person we can change is ourselves, that is why God gave us agency.

Dr. Lund continues " I realize that my energies are best spent on developing my skills to coexist with emotional porcupines and not on changing them." Changing yourself is an independent goal. Trying to change someone else is a wish."

Chapter 3

PEACE

―――――――――――――

As we study the scriptures we see that righteous men and woman had trials, challenges, and heartaches. Were they happy 24 hours a day? If happiness is defined as having no problems, no worries, or difficulties, then we could probably say that they were not happy all the time. Yet perhaps another definition of happiness would be better. INNER PEACE!!!

Through our earth life experience we will have much conflict as we strive to have our spirit learn to control our emotions and our physical body and as we learn to be more Christ like. To not be angry, to forgive, and to love.

We wanted to gain a physical body so that we could if we lived righteously return to Heavenly Father, and have a fulness of Joy. So the experiences gained from earth life can be stepping stones to eternal happiness. The gospel has the saving ordinances. Baptism is the gateway, temple marriage is our goal, so that husband and wife and families can be sealed together forever.

Elder Robert D. Hales of the Quorum of the twelve Apostles in Ensign, September 2011 "A Little Heaven on Earth" Pg 45   "*Temple marriage* describes the place you go to have a marriage performed. *Celestial marriage* is what you create by being true to the sacred covenants you make during the temple marriage ceremony.

"If we live the laws pertaining to celestial marriage, we will, with our spouse and with our family, be able to have a little heaven on earth. And when we live those laws, we are practicing the same laws that are practiced in heaven. We are practicing how to live with the Father and the Son and with our families in the eternities to come. That to me is the message to the world of the Church of Jesus Christ of Latter-day Saints."

Joseph B. Wirthlin said, "Earth life is a period of probation to provide an opportunity for choices. Two mighty forces are pulling in opposite directions. On the one hand is the power of Christ and his righteousness. On the other hand is Satan and the spirits who follow him. President Marion G. Romney said: "Mankind....must determine to travel in company with the one or the other. The reward for following the one is the fruit of the Spirit------peace. The reward for following the other is the works of the flesh--the antithesis of peace." Further he said: "The price of peace is victory over Satan." (Ensign, Oct. 1983, pp. 4,5) We can know which one to follow because God has given everyone the Spirit of Christ to know good from evil and to protect themselves from sin. (See Moro. 7:15-18) We sometimes refer to the Spirit of Christ as our conscience. If we follow its promptings, we can be free of sin and filled with peace. If we do not, but instead let our carnal appetites control us, we never will know true peace." (Ensign, May 1991, "Peace Within", Joseph B. Wirthlin

PLANT YOUR OWN GARDEN
(Pull out the weeds while they are LITTLE)

Positive attitude is so important and helps, being able to see what is good. In order to have a beautiful garden you need to first of all decide what you want to grow. Get your garden spot ready with soil, fertilizer, have your seeds ready, and plant. Then tend your garden, water, weed, what ever it needs. As your garden begins to grow you have all these positive thoughts of picking the vine ripened tomatoes. You can almost taste the fresh picked corn steaming from just being cooked with the melting butter on top. You visualize it bringing forth it's yummy produce. You have a watering system that allows you to leave and not have to worry about the plants getting dry. You see that each section is up and growing as it should. Then work, family, other things take a high priority, even though you know you should check your garden , you know it will be fine because of your positive attitude, it now becomes weeks since you have even looked at it. Deciding to take a look and see the progress over the last several weeks, you step outside and are horrified because all you see is this big jungle of vines and tall plants that you didn't plant and can't even recognize.

1 Nephi 17:1,2,,5 Chapter 16: 35 & 36   You have to recognize your weeds, and pull them out or they will over take your garden , You can't just say, there are no weeds, no weeds, You need to find out what the stuffed emotion or feeling is, is it anger, hurt, sadness,, what happened to cause you to feel this way, stuffing it is saying there are NO WEEDS. Feelings have vibrations, it is energy, energy can't be erased, or just vanish, but it can be transformed or changed from negative to positive. Go over what you really feel.

While in the Garden of Eden, the Lord told Adam and Eve that this life would be hard and that they would learn from their own experience good from evil. So as we also are learning from trial and error, pain, an sorrow, the Lord said in John 14:16-18,27

"And I will pray the Father, and he shall give you another Comforter, that he may abide with you for ever; Even the Sprit of truth; whom the world cannot receive, because it seeth him not, neither knoweth him; but ye know him; for he dwelleth with you, and shall be in you. I will not leave you comfortless; I will come to you."

"PEACE I LEAVE WITH YOU, MY PEACE I GIVE UNTO YOU; NOT AS THE WORLD GIVETH, GIVE I UNTO YOU. Let not your heart be troubled, neither let it be afraid."

In the *Doctrine and Covenants, Student Manual*, page 73,

"Shortly before he was crucified, Jesus promised his disciples the gift of peace (see John 14:27). This peace is not the peace of the world but the inner peace that comes from the knowledge that one has found the truth, and has had his sins remitted, and is on the path that leads to eternal life. This knowledge and assurance comes from the Holy Ghost, who is appropriately called the Comforter (see John 14:26). Thus, all Saints may in this world of strife and turmoil receive peace from Christ by the Holy Ghost and the assurance that the course they are pursuing is correct." (see D&C 6:22-23; 59:23).

John 14:27 "Peace I leave with you, my peace I give unto you; not as the world giveth, give I unto you. Let not your heart be troubled, neither let it be afraid."

"There are laws that govern peace, despite the circumstances, environment, or condition of our lives. When we learn, understand and obey those laws, we inherit the natural consequences of obedience to them, namely peace. When we obey those laws, no one and nothing can take the peace from our hearts." (Art E. Berg, "Finding Peace in Troubled Waters")

D. & C. 130: 20,21 explain this "There is a law, irrevocably decreed in heaven before the foundations of this world, upon which all blessings are predicated— And when we obtain any blessing from God, it is by obedience to that law upon which it is predicated." As man thinketh in his heart, so is he (Prov. 23:7) Our thoughts determine the direction we will go, just as a horse if you pull the reins to the right he will go that direction. Your thoughts and your focus set the course you will take.

President Marion G. Romney, said, "The great overall struggle in the world today is, as it has always been, for the souls of men. Every soul is personally engaged in the struggle, and he makes his fight with what is in his mind. In the final analysis the battleground is, for each individual, within himself. Inevitably he gravitates toward the subjects of his thoughts.. . . . .

"If we would escape the lusts of the flesh and build for ourselves and our children great and noble characters, we must keep in our minds and in their minds true and righteous principles for our thoughts and their thoughts to dwell upon. . . . . .

"I am persuaded, my brothers and sisters, that it is irrational to hope to escape the lusts of the world without substituting for them as the subjects of our thoughts the things of the Spirit.
(In Conference Report, Apr. 1980, pp. 88-89; or Ensign, May 1980 Pp. 66-67.)

There is a Primary song, "Keep the Commandments" Written by Barbara A. McConochie. "Keep the commandments;   keep the commandments! In this there is safety; in this there is peace. He will send blessings; He will send blessings. Words of a prophet;   Keep the commandments. In this there is safety and peace. In this there is safety and peace."
(Barbara A. McConochie *Children's Song Book*, pg 136,137)

As it says in D.&C. 59:23 , "But learn that he who doeth the works of righteousness shall receive his reward, even peace in this world, and eternal life in the world to come."
And to make it have even more impact verse 23, "I, the Lord have spoken it, and the Spirit beareth record. Amen"

What a marvelous promise from the Lord, this great inner peace, brings such comfort.

President John Taylor said, "Peace is the gift of God. Do you want peace? Go to God. Do you want peace in your families? Go to God. Do you want peace to brood over your families? If you do, live your religion, and the very peace of God will dwell and abide with you, for that is where

46

peace comes from, and it [does not] dwell anywhere else."

"Some, in speaking of war and troubles, will say, are you not afraid? No, I am a servant of God, and this is enough, for Father is at the helm. It is for me to be as clay in the hands of the potter, to be pliable and walk in the light of the countenance of the Spirit of the Lord, and then no matter what comes. Let the lightnings flash and the earthquakes bellow, God is at the helm, and I feel like saying but little, for the Lord God Omnipotent reigneth and will continue his work until he has put all enemies under his feet, and his kingdom extends from the rivers to the ends of the earth." JOHN TAYLOR "Teachings of Presidents of the Church" , pg. 150

John 16:33 "These things I have spoken unto you, that in me ye might have peace. In the world ye shall have tribulation: but be of good cheer: I have overcome the world."

President Gordon B. Hinckley said, "Peace may be denied for a season. . . . . . .But God our Eternal Father will watch over this nation and all of the civilized world who look to Him. . . . . .Our safety lies in repentance. Our strength comes from obedience to the commandments of God.

"Are these perilous times? They are. But there is no need to fear. We can have peace in our hearts and peace in our homes. We can be an influence for good in this world, every one of us." (From an October 2001 general conference address). The New Era, November 2001

Joseph B. Wirthlin, said, "Despite dismal conditions in the world and the personal challenges that come into every life, peace within can be a reality. We can be calm and serene regardless of the swirling turmoil all about us. Attaining harmony within our selves depends upon our relationship with our Savior and Redeemer, Jesus Christ, and our willingness to emulate him by living the principles he has given us." Joseph B. Wirthlin   "Peace Within" Ensign May 1991, pg 38

47

The Lord will help us as we draw closer to Him and as we strive to live righteously. King Benjamin tells his people of the great rewards of keeping the commandments.

Mosiah 2:41 "And moreover, I would desire that ye should consider on the BLESSED AND HAPPY STATE OF THOSE THAT KEEP THE COMMANDMENTS OF GOD. For behold, they are blessed in all things, both temporal and spiritual; and if they hold out faithful to the end they are received into heaven, that thereby they may DWELL WITH GOD IN A STATE OF NEVER ENDING   HAPPINESS."

The scriptures are true. As we hold on to the iron rod in faithfulness ,   THE TIME WILL COME WHEN - -- - -   WE WILL DWELL WITH GOD IN A STATE OF NEVER-ENDING HAPPINESS!!!!

President George Q. Cannon stated, "Whenever darkness fills our minds, we may know that we are not possessed of the Spirit of God, and we must get rid of it. When we are filled with the Spirit of God, we are filled with joy, with peace and with happiness no matter what our circumstances may be; for it is a spirit of cheerfulness and of happiness." (George Q. Cannon *Gospel Truth*, 1:19-20)

Elder Jeffrey R. Holland said, "Yes, peace is a very precious commodity, a truly heartfelt need, and there are many things we can do to achieve it. But-----for whatever reason---life has its moments when uninterrupted peace may seem to elude us for a season. We may wonder why there are such times in life, particularly when we may be trying harder than we have ever tried to live worthy of God's blessings and obtain His help. When problems of sorrows or sadness come and they *don't* seem to be our fault, what are we to make of their unwelcome appearance?"

"With time and perspective we recognize that such problems in life do come for a purpose, if only to allow the one who faces such despair to be convinced that he really does need divine strength beyond himself, that she really does need the offer of heaven's hand. Those who feel no need for mercy usually never seek it and almost never bestow it. Those who have never had a heartache or a weakness or felt lonely or forsaken never have had to cry unto heaven for relief of such personal pain. Surely it is better to find the goodness of God and the grace of Christ, even at the price of despair, than to risk living our lives in a moral or material complacency that has never felt any need for faith or forgiveness, any need for redemption or relief."

"A life without problems or limitations or challenges---life without opposition in all thing---as Lehi phrased it- - - - - -would be less rewarding and less ennobling. - - - - - - - -As beloved Eve said, were it not for the difficulties faced in a fallen world, neither she nor Adam nor any of the rest of us ever would have known "the joy of our redemption, and the eternal life which God giveth unto all the obedient." Moses 5:11

"So life has its oppositions and its conflicts, and the gospel of Jesus Christ has answers and assurances."   Jeffrey R. Holland *Ensign*, November 1996, pg. 83-84

President Howard W. Hunter said, "Whenever Jesus lays his hands upon lives, if Jesus lays his hands upon a marriage, it lives. If he is allowed to lay his hands on the family, it lives."
(Howard W. Hunter *Conference Report*, Oct. 1979, 93.)

Plant your garden, but be sure and pull out the weeds

1. Recognize the weeds   you need to know what they are

2. You can give the garden plenty of water, and lots of things will grow, including the weeds, what are the weeds, they are negative thinking.

49

3. Mourn - - - if something truly bothers you, it is very important to not just stuff it. How do you handle it, just say I'm HAPPY , I'm Happy. I have tried that. One time one of my children thought I did not help as much as I should have. Years ago , I figured that I should just let it go, I tried, but it was still niggling at me, I kept saying "I'm Happy , I should not let this bother me, finally I told my husband , He graciously listened, I went on for about 30 min, and he just listened , After this time, I felt so much better, I was able to get it out recognize it and move forward. I had to examine it. Was this a plant, or was it a weed in disguise. It was not something I needed to hang on to. The weed was there. It did hurt. It was real, but by looking at it and saying "Oh this is really a weed, a dandelion that I don't want in my garden , I will pull it out and move on.

Not everything is so easy, sometimes there is a huge boulder and it takes, many prayers and the help of the Savior to forgive, as you work around it. And plant flowers around it.

Our daughter Larissa felt very impressed for several years that there were 2 girls that were to be part of their family. They already had 3 boys and 1 girl, and wanted more but she wasn't able to get pregnant again. These 2 girls came to her in a dream and let her know they would be coming a different way. They thought perhaps adoption, so they registered with several agencies. Nothing happened, they thought perhaps foster care. Beautiful children came to their home, even twin boys to be taken care of by them, they loved them all, yet each time they felt these were not the ones.

About 2 years after Larissa's dream, the agency asked if they would care for 3 children, 2 girls and a boy. Karen only 6 months, Jaden 2, and Jarith 3. They talked it over with their family, their oldest 15 and the youngest 6. They all agreed and after meeting the kids they all hoped they could adopt them.

The birth parents of these children were on drugs and had many issues. The children were left with relatives often and the kids felt abandoned. They felt the love of Larissa's family, and soon were calling them mommy and daddy.

The 3 year old would hop on Larissa's lap put her arms around her and say "Mommie, I love you."   She did this over and over. I was able to watch the love that the children were being shown, and the love they gave back. But, it was not to be. The children had to go back.

WATCH THE WEATHER (BE PREPARED, CARRY AN UMBRELLA

And your own SUNSHINE.

The weather fore-cast lets us know if it is supposed to be clear, rainy, snowy, high winds, etc. We prepare by bringing our sun-screen if it is hot and we are going to the beach. If it predicts rain, we bring our umbrella. Like wise , if it is cold and perhaps snow, we wear or bring our warmest coat, mittens , snow boots, hat. Anything we can do to prepare and protect ourselves.

How can we carry our own sunshine if it is raining. We can't change the weather.. We carry it on the inside. We have our umbrella to keep us dry, and we carry a sunshine attitude.

Knowing the things that are going to happen in the last days, which is now, how do we move forward with a positive attitude, even more, how do we move forward.

In 2 Timothy 3:1-5, it tells of a lot of the wickedness,
"This know also, that in the last days perilous times shall come."

Then it goes on to say all of the wickedness that is going on today, we can see it, we can read about it, it is everywhere. Because of this wickedness there will be wars and rumors of wars, famine, earthquakes, storms, it is in indeed perilous times. How do we move without fear. How do we plan ahead.

These following ideas are taken from a talk Barbara Jones gave in 2004 for the B. Y. U. Television channel, a segment entitled "Time for Teens" I watched the rebroadcast 14 of March, 2008 on the B. Y. U. Channel.

Barbara was looking for happiness; a time when everything would be perfect and she would be happy. She went to a school that taught Ballet, which she loved. She noticed the other girls were much trimmer than she was, and seemed to be happy. So she went on a campaign to lose the weight , in time she lost so much weight that she got sick and had to leave the school. Where was the happiness.

Then several years later Barbara saw that her friends were getting married and having families. "That is what I need to do,"   Get married, and then I will have arrived, then I will be happy."

Barbara married a friend of the boy she had dated for many years. She figured, "Yes, now I will be happy , now I have arrived."   However her husband had many problems, he was not mentally balanced and he tried to kill her three different times.

Barbara had gone back to her ballet, and now had a small son. During one of her performances her husband was backstage and beckoned that something was wrong with their son and that she needed to leave immediately. As she met him at the car, he bound her hands and feet and threw her in the truck. After driving for some time he stopped in an isolated place, pulled her out and got his shot gun, he pointed it at her knee and said , "Now you will never dance again."   Barbara was terrified, but she managed a prayer. "God, where are you, please help me."

52

Her husband put the gun back in the car, and drove off leaving her there. He later killed himself.

We are living in the last days, when great wickedness is upon the earth, yet the Lord commands us to be of good cheer.

"Wherefore, be of good cheer and do not fear, for I the Lord am with you, and will stand by you; and ye shall bear record of me, even Jesus Christ, that I am the Son of the living God, that I was, that I am and that I am to come."   D. & C. 68:6

" Verily I say unto you my friends, fear not, let your hearts be comforted; yea, rejoice evermore, and in everything give thanks;" D. & C. 98:1

"- - - - - and all things wherewith you have been afflicted shall work together for your good, and to my name's glory" - - - D. & C. 98:3

"Lift up your head and be of good cheer;" - - - - -3 Nephi 1:13
What an exciting time to live in, the time before the 2nd Coming of our Savior. It is no accident that we are here on the earth at this time. The Lord reserved some of his most Valiant and strong children to be his Righteous Warriors in these latter days.

Mary moved into the house across the street 10 years ago. Her and her husband had accepted the gospel and been sealed in the temple, however for whatever reason they returned to their old habits of smoking and left the church. When they moved in we tried to befriend them and accept them for who they were. We had no idea that they were members of the church. In fact one day they gave us a book which happened to be The Book of Mormon, saying that the previous owners must have left it, but since we were Mormon we could probably use it.

After several years Mary decided to take us up on our invitation to

53

attend church, she became active and even went to the temple again.

Mary had a lot of health problems that got progressively worse. She had diabetics then several strokes, her speech was affected, it was very difficult to understand her.

I don't know what kind of training or upbringing he had but he was always putting down his wife. Very verbally abusive. I would say Mary you look pretty today, and he would say no she doesn't, she's ugly. He was constantly mean to her.

But Mary carried her own sunshine, she would laugh (I'm sure it hurt her) but she just kept trying to go on.

Chapter 4

FAITH

<hr>

FAITH OR FEAR
The choice is ours.

Faith and fear are like opposite sides of a coin. They are like the difference between night and day. Light and darkness cannot exist in the same place at the same time. Faith is of God. Fear is of Satan. In the Garden of Eden Adam and Eve hid themselves because they were afraid.

Moses 4: 14 - 16 And they heard the voice of the Lord God, as they were walking in the garden---and Adam and his wife went to hide themselves from the presence of the Lord God.

And I, the Lord God, called unto Adam, and said unto him: Where goest thou? And he said: I heard thy voice in the garden, and **I WAS AFRAID."**

Adam & Eve had recently encountered Satan and had done as God had forbidden, never the less they still had their agency to choose.

In the Bible Dictionary, pg. 762 it explains fear. "The first effect of Adam's sin was that he was afraid. Sin destroys that feeling of confidence God's child should feel in a loving Father, and produces instead a feeling of shame and guilt. Ever since the Fall, God has been teaching men NOT TO FEAR, but with penitence to ask forgiveness in full confidence of receiving it."

Perhaps this is a major reason Satan wants us to sin------so that we will lose the confidence that we are a child of God. So that we will be fearful to be in His presence.

President James E. Faust, in an article entitled "Be Not Afraid", *Ensign*, October 2002, pg. 3 , said, "Satan is our greatest enemy and works night and day to destroy us. But we need not become paralyzed with fear of Satan's power. He can have no power over us unless we permit it. He is really a coward, and if we stand firm he will retreat."

Where do we find inner peace and confidence? We find it by living the gospel and keeping the commandments of God. Joseph F..Smith stated: "We hear about living in perilous times. We are in perilous times, but I do not feel the pangs of that terror. It is not upon me. I propose to live so that it will not rest upon me. I propose to live so that I shall be immune from the perils of the world, if it be possible for me to so live, by obedience to the commandments of God and to his laws revealed for my guidance. No matter what may come to me, if I am only in the line of my duty, if I am in fellowship with God, if I am worthy of the fellowship of my brethren, if I can stand spotless before the world, without blemish, without transgression of the laws of God, what does it matter to me what may happen to me? I am always ready, if I am in this frame of understanding, mind and conduct. It does not matter at all. Therefore, I borrow no trouble nor feel the pangs of fear." (Joseph F..Smith "The Gospel a Shield from Terror," *Improvement Era*, July 1917, p. 827.}

This statement was made over 90 years ago. We are living in the 2nd Millenium. The wickedness of the world has increased greatly. The sins of Sodom and Gomora are not only being practiced, but openly hailed as an alternate life style that is good. Things that were not mentioned because it was serious sin are now being broadcast on the air waves. The world is now as it was in the days of Noah, perhaps worse because of abortion.

"Wo unto them that call evil good, and good evil, that put darkness for light, and light for darkness, that put bitter for sweet, and sweet for bitter!" 2 Nephi 15:20

Bishop Keith B. McMullin (Second Counselor in the Presiding Bishopric) in "The New Era", February 2003, page 38 stated: "Satan is real and is on the earth as well. He and his legions are wreaking havoc among the children of men. He speaks no truth, feels no love, promotes no good, and avows nothing but mayhem and destruction."

As Bishop Keith B. McMullin explains the Lord warns us, especially in D.& C. 1:35

"For I am no respecter of persons, and will that all men shall know that the day speedily cometh; the hour is not yet, but is nigh at hand, when peace shall be taken from the earth, and the devil shall have power over his own dominion."

Bishop McMullin goes on to say, ------- "peace has now been taken from the earth, and the devil has power over his dominion. His beguiling ways are mesmerizing the people. Temptation is on every hand. Crassness and wrangling have become a way of life. What was once considered awful is now considered tame; what at first titillates, soon captivates and then destroys."

I remember my mother telling me when I was a teenager to not look at or read certain magazines These were what you would call trashy things that no self respecting person would look at. They were not pornography   they were just articles on how "other people lived." These other people's life style were not in harmony with gospel teachings. Even years ago when the world seemed to be more innocent, you may occasionally overhear, peers talking about this or that. Now today, it is shocking to hear what is on the news, things I didn't even know existed,

Immorality is flaunted , as opposite sex attraction is also. What used to go on behind hidden doors, is now out in the open, magazines lining the checkout counter of the grocery story have pictures of scantily clothed women , and highlighted articles of unfaithfulness of famous people. It is no longer a sly suggestion , it is broadcast openly.

President Boyd K. Packer in a meeting Feb. 28, 2004 to members of the J. Reuben Clark Law Society, given in the Conference Center theater and as written in *the Church News*, 6 March 2004, page 5. Entitled "Defend the faith". President Packer said, "the world is spiraling downward at an ever-quickening pace. I am sorry to tell you that it will not get better."

"Nothing happened in Sodom and Gomorrah which exceeds the wickedness and depravity which surrounds us now.

"Satan uses every intrigue to disrupt the family. The sacred relationship between man and woman, husband and wife, through which mortal bodies are conceived and life is passed from one generation to the next generation, is being showered with filth.

"Profanity, vulgarity, blasphemy, and pornography are broadcast into the homes and minds of the innocent. Unspeakable wickedness, perversion, and abuse------not even exempting little children-----once hidden in dark places, now seeks protection from courts and judges."

President Packer told the worldwide audience that others will look to them for legal counsel. "You have, or should have, the spirit of discernment. It was given you when you had conferred upon you the gift of the holy Ghost. You must locate where the snares are hidden and help guide our footsteps around them."

President Packer said the world is now where ancient prophets warned it would be.

"Paul prophesied word by word and phrase by phrase, describing things exactly as they are now," he said. "I quote from Paul's prophecy and check the words that fit our society. . . . ."

"For men shall be lovers of their own selves - - -check!

Covetous - - - -check!

Proud----check!

Blasphemers ----check!

Disobedient to parents - - -check! Check!

Unthankful - - --check!

Unholy - - -check!

Without natural affection - - check!

Trucebreakers - - -check!

False accusers - - - - check!

Incontinent - - - check!

Fierce - - - - - check!

Despisers of those that are good - - - -check!

Traitors - - - - - check!

Heady - - - -check!

High-minded - - - - check!

Lovers of pleasures more than lovers of God -check! Check!

Quoting Brigham Young and Joseph Smith, President Packer said even in the worst times the United States Constitution will not be destroyed, but "this people will step forth and save it from the threatened destruction."

" I do not know when that day will come or how it will come to pass," said President Packer. "I feel sure that when it does come to pass, among those who will step forward from among this people will be men who hold the Holy Priesthood and who carry as credentials a bachelor or doctor of law degree. And women, also, of honor. And there will be judges, as well.

"Others from the world outside the Church will come, as Colonel Thomas Kane did, and bring with them their knowledge of the law to protect this people.

"We may one day stand alone, but we will not change or lower our standards or change our course. "

President Wilford Woodruff declared: "God has held the angels of destruction for many years, lest they should reap down the wheat with the tares. But I want to tell you now, that those angels have left the portals of heaven, and they stand over this people and this nation now, and are hovering over the earth waiting to pour out the judgments. And from this very day they shall be poured out. Calamities and troubles are increasing in the earth, there is a meaning to these things. Remember this, and reflect upon these matters. If you do your duty and I do my duty, we'll have protection, and shall pass through the afflictions in peace and in safety. (Young Women's Journal, Aug. 1894, pp. 512-13)

Elder Orson Pratt said,
     - - - "Then the servants of God will need to be armed with the power of God, they will need to have that sealing blessing pronounced upon their foreheads that they can stand forth in the midst of these desolations and plagues and not be overcome by them" - - - -Another angel ascended from the east and cried to the four angels, and said, 'Smite not the earth now, but wait a little while' How long?' 'Until the servants of our God are sealed in their foreheads" What for ? To prepare them to stand forth in the midst of these desolations and plagues, and not be overcome. When they are prepared, when they have received a renewal of their bodies in the Lord's temple, and have been filled with the holy Ghost and purified as gold and silver in a furnace of fire, then they will be prepared to stand before the nations of the earth and preach glad tidings of salvation in the midst of judgments that are to come like a whirlwind upon the wicked."   (Orson Pratt, *Journal of Discourses*, 15:365-66)   *D.& C. Study guide* p. 179

By going to Gods Holy House, by keeping our covenants, by honoring the Priesthood the Lord will help us. As Nephi saw in our latter days, the saints will be armed with righteousness and with the power of God.

"And it came to pass that I, Nephi, beheld the power of the Lamb of God, that it descended upon the saints of the church of the Lamb, and upon the covenant people of the Lord, who were scattered upon all the face of the earth; and they were armed with righteousness and with the power of God in great glory."

1 Nephi 14:14

Elder David E. Sorensen said,
"The temple is a place of revelation, of inspiration, mediation, and peace--- a place to restore ourselves, to clear our minds, to find answers to our prayers, and to enjoy the satisfaction of worship and service." (David E. Sorensen, *Ensign*, Oct. 2003
'The Doctrine of Temple Work' pg. 36)

The Lord saved some of his most valiant children for these the last days, to help prepare the Kingdom of God for the Savior's coming. But Satan's powers has also been unleashed. The forces for good and evil are rallying. We have to choose to follow Christ, because, if we sit by and don't choose, we choose by default. Because Satan is ever ready and willing to have the channels of our mind lose the guiding beam of the Lord, and listen to his voice.

President Boyd K. Packer in a meeting to Church Educational System educators, (gathered in the Salt Lake Tabernacle on the 6th of February, 2004, and as written in the *Church News* 14 February 2004 "Teaching Faith"   Pg. 5) , said "I know of nothing in the history of the Church or in the world to compare with our present circumstances. Nothing happened in Sodom and Gomorrah which exceeds in wickedness and depravity that which surrounds us now."

"Words of profanity, vulgarity, and blasphemy are heard everywhere. Unspeakable wickedness and perversion were once hid in dark places; now they are in the open, even accorded legal protection. At Sodom and Gomorrah these things were localized, Now they are spread across the world, and they are among us."

"The one pure defense"----a knowledge and testimony of the gospel of Jesus Christ.

President Packer said he came before the teachers as did Jacob when he taught in the temple "having first obtained mine errand from the Lord." Jacob 1:17

"Teach your students of the Apostasy and the Restoration of the priesthood, of Joseph Smith and the organization of The church of Jesus Christ of Latter-day Saints, by the Lord's own declaration, 'the only true and living church upon the face of the whole earth'   D.& C. 1:30 Immerse them in the truths of the Book of Mormon. That will lead them to the truth and to the promise that is there, and then they will be armed with the protective influence of the truth."

With an individual testimony, he said, young people today will be safe in the world.

"The world is spiraling downward at an ever quickening pace. I am sorry to tell you that it will not get better. "It is my purpose to charge each of you as teachers with the responsibility---to put you on alert. These are days of great spiritual danger for our youth." "Spiritual diseases of epidemic proportions sweep over the world. We are not able to curb them. But we can prevent our youth from being infected by them.

"Knowledge and a testimony of the restored gospel of Jesus 'Christ are like a vaccine. We can inoculate them. "Inoculate: In--'to be

within' and occulate means 'eye to see.'   We place an eye within them--the unspeakable gift of the Holy Ghost. Young people need not
fear. Their teachers need not fear. Fear is the opposite of faith. I have been in the councils of the Church and seen many things. I have seen disappointment and shock and concern. Never once have I seen any fear.

"Our youth can look forward with hope for a happy life. They
shall marry and raise families in the Church and teach their little ones what you have taught them. They, in turn will teach their children
and their grandchildren." Elder M. Russell Ballard of the
Quorum of the twelve Apostles, in an article M. Russell Ballard, "Preparing for the Future," *Ensign* September 2011 page 28

"Faith is a principle of the Gospel. Faith is one of the greatest
powers that you and I have in this sojourn of mortality. Fear is one of
those principles that the devil uses. He likes to seed in your minds and in mine doubt and question. He's the father of all lies; he lies to us, and he can confuse us if we allow ourselves to be caught up in fear. So replace any fear or apprehension you have now with faith---faith in the Lord Jesus Christ, faith in your fathers and your mothers. Stay close to them."

As our son Seth Sinclair wrote to us while on his mission in
Paraguay. " The forces of evil and good seem to be accelerating. People are rushing by so quickly, whether doing work for the Lord or for Satan, that their impact knocks the fence sitters off the fence."
Who's side are we on. Do we have a firm grip on the iron rod, which is the word of God. Do we study from the scriptures daily. Do we read, and meditate to learn God's word. We have challenges, and problems, do we realize that in the scriptures we can find the answers.

"feast upon the words of Christ; for behold, the words of Christ
will tell you all things what ye should do." 2 Nephi 32:3

Do we realize the great blessings that are in store for us. President Benson gave great promises to us, if we would read the Book of Mormon. "There is a power in the book which will begin to flow into your lives the moment you begin a serious study of the book. You will find power to resist temptation, to avoid deception, and you will find power to stay on the strait and narrow path."

"And those who receive it in faith and work righteousness, shall receive a crown of eternal life;" D.&C. 20:14

President James E. Faust , "A Priceless Heritage", July, *Ensign* 2002, page 6 stated,
"The faithful members, with all their faults and failings, are humbly striving to do God's holy work across the world. We need your help in the great struggle against the powers of darkness so prevalent in the world today. - - - - - - You can have great meaning and purpose in your lives, even in the profane world in which we live. You can have strength of character so that you can act for yourselves and not be acted upon." (See 2 Nephi 2:26)

We live in very wicked times, yet the Lord has told us , Be of Good Cheer and do not fear for I the Lord am with you and will stand by you--, D. & C. 68:6.

How can we possible have faith in such a troubled world? God knows all things, he knows the end from the beginning. This is His plan. "But the Lord knoweth all things from the beginning; wherefore, he prepareth a way to accomplish all his works among the children of men; for behold, he hath all power unto the fulfilling of all his words." 1 Nephi 9:6

Just consider the plan of Satan to stop the Book of Mormon from coming forth by having a snare so tight with the 116 pages of manuscript that was translated from the first part of the Book of Mormon. Martin

Harris begged Joseph Smith to ask the Lord if he could show them, to his wife and a few others. Twice the Lord said no, yet Martin persisted. Joseph asked again and the Lord said yes, but was very strict in who he could show them to. Martin broke his commitment and the pages were lost.

The Lord taught a very important lesson to the young prophet, which all of us need to learn and apply.

"For, behold, you should not have feared man more than God Although men set at naught the counsels of God, and despise his words.

"Yet you should have been faithful; and he would have extended his arm and supported you against all the fiery darts of the adversary; *and he would have been with you in every time of trouble."* D. & C. 3:7,8.

Elder Joseph B. Wirthlin said, "Our Father in Heaven does not want us to cower. He does not want us to wallow in our misery. He expects us to square our shoulders, roll up our sleeves, and overcome our challenges."

"That kind of spirit---that blend of faith and hard work---is the spirit we should emulate as we seek to reach a safe harbor in our own lives.

"Use your ingenuity, your strength, your might to resolve your challenges. Do all you can do and then leave the rest to the Lord." (Joseph B. Wirthlin "Finding a Safe Harbor, *"Ensign*, May 2000, pg 60-61)

Elder Richard G. Scott said, "Your trust in the Lord must be more powerful and enduring than your confidence in your own personal feelings and experience."

"To exercise faith is to trust that the Lord Knows what He is doing with you and that He can accomplish it for your eternal good even though you cannot understand how He can possibly do it. We are like infants in our understanding of eternal matters and their impact on us here in mortality. Yet at times we act as if we knew it all. When you pass through trials for His purposes, as you trust Him, exercise faith in Him, He will help you. That support will generally come step by step, a portion at a

time. While you are passing through each phase, the pain and difficulty that comes from being enlarged will continue. If all matters were immediately resolved at your first petition, you could not grow." (Richard G. Scott, "Trust in the Lord," Ensign, Nov. 1995, pg 17).

Faith in God, trusting Him completely, what a learning process that is. At times that is very difficult, we do not know the answers we do the best we can with our limited knowledge, and wonder how can God completely know our situation "But God you don't understand. My thinking is the right answer, this is what I want, and I want it now."

In D. & C. 78: 17, 18, 19 God answers this question. "Verily, verily, I say unto you, ye are little children, and ye have not as yet understood how great blessings the Father hath in his own hands and prepared for you. And ye cannot "bear all things now; nevertheless, be of good cheer for I will lead you along. The kingdom is yours and the blessings there of are yours, and the riches of eternity are yours.

"And he who receiveth all things with thankfulness shall be made glorious; and the things of this earth shall be added unto him, even an hundred fold, yea, more."

Elder Neal A. Maxwell said, "Patient endurance permits us to cling to our faith in the Lord and our faith in His timing when we are being tossed about by the surf of circumstance. Even when a seeming undertow grasps us, somehow, in the tumbling, we are being carried forward." (Ensign, May 1990, pg. 34)

Then in D. & C. 10, the Lord explains the plans of Satan and how he inspired wicked men. Verse 20, Verily, verily, I say unto you, that Satan has great hold upon their hearts; he stirreth them up to iniquity against that which is good.

Verse 33 Thus Satan thinketh to overpower your testimony in this generation, that the work may not come forth in this generation.

Verse 43 I will not suffer that they shall destroy my work; yea, I will show unto them that my wisdom is greater than the cunning of the devil.

The Lord knows all things, he placed you on the earth at this time and place because you were valiant in the pre-existence. He knows your strengths. He knows you and loves you. In 2nd Nephi 9:20 as Jacob is talking to his family . . . . . "O how great the holiness of our God! For he knoweth all things, and there is not anything save he knows it.

President Harold B. Lee said in reference to the above scripture, "Now, if you will just keep that in mind you have a beginning point, you have a relationship with Him. We are His son, His daughter. He knows us. He knows the very things and the times before appointed, and the place where we would live, and the times in which we would live. So in Him only can we place full trust." (Harold B. Lee, "Teachings of Presidents of the Church", pg.53)

That means if we follow the Lord we will be protected and need not fear. The Lord provided a way for the escape of the children of Israel , when the armies of the Pharo were behind them and the Red Sea before them.

For those who would repent they could have been on the boat with Noah. The Lord does provide the way if we will listen to his prophets and follow their counsel, and part of that is daily prayer and scripture study.

We live in a time of great wickedness. Elder Richard G. Scott at a BYU-Idaho devotional February 24, 2004 said "The world is being engulfed in a rising river of degenerate filth, with the abandonment of virtue, righteousness, traditional marriage, family life and personal integrity. President Hinckley has warned publicly that conditions are comparable to those of Sodom and Gomorrah, the epitome of unholy life in the Old Testament."

Continuing Elder Scott said, "Satan skillfully manipulates the power of media and other channels of communication. We cannot dry up the mounting river of evil influences for they are the result of the exercise of moral agency divinely granted by our Father to His children. But we can, with clarity, warn of the consequences of getting close to its enticing, devouring current. We can even provide life preservers for those caught in those vanquishing waters who recognize the need for help."

" God has provided a way to live in this world and not be contaminated by the degrading pressures evil agents spread through it. .You can live a virtuous, productive, righteous life by following the plan of protection created by your Father in Heaven, It is contained in the scriptures and in the inspired declarations of His prophets. - - - - -When understood and lived, the doctrines they contain powerfully motivate uplifting righteous behavior despite worldly decay. Our Father in Heaven knows His children. He knew that many would choose the wrong paths and that our period would be flooded with temptations of every order and iniquity in every corner. He also knew how you can live successfully in that environment. His scriptures tell you how it is done."
(Church News 28 February 2004, 'Plan of Protection' pg. 7)

"Therefore, whosoever belongeth to my church need not fear, for such shall inherit the kingdom of heaven."   D.& C. 10:55

"And now, behold, whosoever is of my church, and endureth of my church to the end, him will I establish upon my rock, and the gates of hell shall not prevail against them." D. & C. 10:69

We need to learn to recognize when the Lord is speaking to us, the promtings of the Spirit. President Harold B. Lee, said "The most important thing you can do is to learn to talk to God. Talk to Him as you would talk to your father, for He is your Father, and He wants you to talk to Him. He wants you to cultivate ears to listen, when He gives you the impressions of the Spirit to tell you what to do. *If you learn to give heed to the sudden ideas which come to your minds, you will find those things coming through in the very hour of your need.* If you will cultivate an ear to hear these promptings, you will have learned to walk by the spirit of revelation.? Itialics and bold added. (Harold B. Lee, *The Teachings of Presidents of the Church*, pg. 55)

President James E Faust said, "Let us not take counsel from our fears. May we remember always to be of good cheer, put our faith in God, and live worthy for Him to direct us. We are each entitled to receive personal inspiration to guide us through our mortal probation. May we so live that our hearts are open at all times to the whisperings and comfort of the Spirit. James E Faust, *Ensign* Oct. 2002, 'Be Not Afraid', pg.6

One of the great tests of our faith is when we lose a loved one. Especially our companion, or a child. Why is a mother of small children taken, they need her so much, her direction, guidance and love. Why is a righteous husband and father taken in the prime of life. What could possibly be more important then his providing for and helping to rear his family. His lovely wife is left with the sole responsibility of providing shelter and food and will probably need to go into the work world.

Doesn't God understand these people are needed here more than on the other side. Elder Neal A. Maxwell said,"Remember Brigham Young's statement about faith in Jesus' character, in Jesus' Atonement, and in the plan of salvation? Such faith should help us more than it is allowed to do by us at times. We can also understand that as important as our labors here are, they have to be put in perspective in the context of that plan."

Elder Maxwell goes on to say, "We do not control what I call "the great transfer board in the sky." The inconveniences that are sometimes associated with release from our labors here are necessary in order to accelerate the work there. Heavenly Father can't do His work there, with 10 times more people than we have on this planet, without on occasion taking some of the very best sisters and brothers from among us. The conditions of termination here, painful though they are, are a part of the conditions of acceleration there. Thus we are back to faith in the timing of God, and to our need to be able to say "Thy *timing* be done," even when we do not fully understand it. Elder Neal A. Maxwell, *Ensign*, July 2002, "The Holy Ghost: Glorifying Christ" pg.61

Elder Lance B. Wickman in October Conference 2002 explained how difficult it was for his family to lose their 5 year old boy Adam. He got a common childhood illness that seemed to be mild, but one morning he would not wake up, he was in a coma. In the hospital the doctors and nurses did everything they could. There were priesthood blessings given , fervent prayers and fasting, yet Adam did not recover.

Elder Wickman states, "I believe that mortality's supreme test is to face the "why" and then let it go, trusting humbly in the Lord's promise that "all things must come to pass in their time." (D&C 64:32).

Elder Wickman explains, "But the Lord has not left us comfortless or with out any answers. As to the healing of the sick, He has clearly said: "And again, it shall come to pass that he that hath faith in me to be healed, *and is not appointed unto death*, shall be healed" (D&C 42:48; emphasis added}. All to often we overlook the qualifying phrase "and is not appointed unto death" ("or," we might add, "unto sickness or handicap". Please do not despair when fervent prayers have been offered and priesthood blessings performed and your loved one makes no improvement or even passes from mortality. Take comfort in the knowledge that you did everything you could. Such faith, fasting, and blessing could not be in vain! That your child did not recover in spite of all that was done in his behalf can and should be the basis for peace and reassurance to all who love him! *The Lord----who inspires the blessings and who hears every earnest prayer---called him home nonetheless.* All the experiences of prayer, fasting, and faith may well have been more for *our* benefit than for his. Lance B. Wickman, *Ensign*, 2002, pg 30,31}

We need to have faith in all areas of our life, in everything the Lord asks us to do. Consider Nephi when the Lord commanded him to build a ship. Had Nephi ever built a boat before? I don't know, but if he had this one would be entirely different because the Lord was the architect. Consider what most of us would say. "I don't know how, I have never done this before."   That would probably be our first response. If we got past that one, then the next major problem, O.K. Lord just give me a couple of years to return to Jerusalem and there I will purchase the tools and come back and begin building.

The faith of Nephi. Oh to have the faith of Nephi. He didn't argue, he didn't say he didn't know how, all he said was,

"Lord, whither shall I go that I may find ore to molten, that I may make tools to construct the ship after the manner which thou hast shown unto me?"   1 Nephi 17:9

Then Nephi went to work , He took the skins of beast and made a bellows, so he could get the fire hot enough to melt the ore and make the tools. He didn't even have a match to start the fire, but said "I did smite two stones together that I might make fire."
1 Nephi 17:11

Was Satan happy that they would have a ship to go to the promised land. Laman and Lemuel who took delight in listening to the adversary, called Nephi a fool ,

71

"And when my brethren saw that I was about to build a ship, they began to murmur against me, saying: Our brother is a fool, for he thinketh that he can build a ship; yea, and he also thinketh that he can cross these great waters."

If that happened to us would our faith be shaken? His two older brothers didn't think he could do it and refused to help. Would we go back to the Lord and say, O.K. Lord, I tried but you know I can't build this ship alone and my brothers won't help. Besides my feeling are hurt and you know how violent Laman and Lemuel can be, remember the times they beat me, and tied me up and were going to kill me.

Nephi didn't quit, he didn't stop , he knew the Lord would show him how and prepare the way even with the great conflict of his brothers Laman and Lemuel..

Nephi does everything he can to help his brothers have faith. He tells them about Moses and the children of Israel. How through the power of God the Red Sea was parted. And many other miracles of the Lord.

"And now, if the Lord has such great power, and has wrought so many miracles among the children of men , **How is it that he cannot instruct me, that I should build a ship?"**
1 Nephi 17:51

Laman and Lemuel were so angry that again they tried to kill Nephi.

"When I had spoken these words they were angry with me, and were desirous to throw me into the depths of the sea; and as they came forth to lay their hands upon me I spake unto them, saying:" In the name of the Almighty God, I command you that ye touch me not, for I am filled with the power of God----- and whoso shall lay his hands upon me shall wither even as a dried reed; and he shall be as naught before the power of God, for God shall smite him." 1Nephi 17:48

Nephi never doubted. He knew the Lord had commanded him to build a ship and that he would open the way.

Our Prophet President Hinckley said "I too believe that God will always make a way where there is no way. I believe that if we will walk in obedience to the commandments of God, if we will follow the counsel of the Priesthood, He will open a way even where there appears to be no way. {Ensign July 1995, 2}

President Boyd K. Packer said in April General Conference, 2000, "We need not live in fear of the future. We have every reason to rejoice and little reason to fear. If we follow the promptings of the Spirit, we will be safe, whatever the future holds. We will be shown what to do. It is a glorious time to live!   No matter what trials await us, we . . . . . and those we love will be guided and corrected and protected and we will be comforted."

What marvelous counsel from, President Packer. We do live in a world that is spiraling down hill at break neck speed. We have been warned and forewarned, by God. But as we keep the commandments we can move forward in faith. God will guide, direct, and protect us. God is telling us to - fear not!.

Elder Tad R. Callister (of the Seventy) has a wonderful article in the *Ensign*, Dec. 2010, "Fear Not" pg. 42-44 Elder Callister tells of the great faith Mary, the mother of Jesus had, when she was told she would have the Son of God. How could this be possible , how would Joseph respond? What would others think?

Mary and Joseph learned early in life that for every problem God has a solution.. To Mary, the angel said: "Fear not . . . For with God

73

nothing shall be impossible."

Reading the prophesies in the scriptures, without having faith that God will protect His people can be very depressing. Wars, rumors of wars, many natural disasters, earthquakes, storms, the waters will be unsafe because Satan will have power over them. Plague, disease, etc. Just listening to the news, or reading the newspaper, with all the anger, rage, mobs. The financial situation, people are losing their jobs, and their homes, unrest where ever you live. We are living in the days as seen by Paul.

"This know also, that in the last days perilous times shall come." 2 Timothy 3:1-5   Then Paul goes on to describe in vivid words, the situation of our world today. Honesty, integrity , morality, are becoming ridiculed. Those who stand for truth and righteousness are criticized.

Paul the Apostle explains Satan's powers, "For we wrestle not against flesh and blood, but against principalities, against powers, against the rulers of the darkness of this world, against spiritual wickedness in high places."   Ephesians 6:12. In the foot notes, it explains the darkness of this world is secret combinations. And that spiritual wickedness in high places is Governments; wickedness.

Still God is looking over his people. One of my favorite scriptures is found in First Nephi :14:14. "And it came to pass that I, Nephi, beheld the power of the Lamb of God, that it descended upon the saints of the church of the Lamb, and upon the covenant people of the Lord, who were scattered upon all the face of the earth; and they were armed with righteousness and with the power of God in great glory. There is our safety. God has a plan, God is in charge.

President Hinckley said, "Let us recognize that fear comes not of God, but rather that this gnawing, destructive element comes from the adversary of truth and righteousness. Fear is the antithesis of faith. It is corrosive in its effects, even deadly;

"For God hath not given us the spirit of fear; but of power, and of love, and of a sound mind." (2 Tim. 1:7)

"We need not fear as long as we have in our lives the power that comes from righteously living by the truth which is from God our Eternal Father. Nor need we fear as long as we have the power of faith." (Ensign, Oct. 1984, 2-3)"

God is there helping us. He knows the way, he is beckoning us to follow him, to look toward him. We are here to walk by faith, and that means putting our trust in him. He tells us so many times and in many different ways, to not fear.

"Fear thou not; for I am with thee: be not dismayed; for I am thy God: I will strengthen thee; yea, I will help thee; yea, I will uphold thee with the right hand of my righteousness." Isaiah 41:10

"For I the Lord thy God will hold thy right hand, saying unto thee, Fear not; I will help thee." Isaiah 41:136

Fear is one of the emotions or feeling we have all experienced in our life. It was with us in the beginning, in Gensis chapter 3:8-10 as Adam and Eve were walking in the garden they heard the voice of the Lord and they hid themselves from the Lord. As God called, "Adam where art thou" "I heard thy voice in the garden, and I was afraid, because I was naked; and I hid myself."

Fear is a feeling we experience when we are in danger, but the Lord says, "Be of Good Cheer, and do not fear, for I the Lord am with you." D. & C. 68:6

In the Ensign, "Make Our House Invisible" August 2011, pages 66, 67 by Alice W. Flade, who lives in Utah, USA. Alice tells of her families experience at the closing of World War II. She was 19 years old and they lived in Europe. Because of the threat of being bombed all the houses were dark because of blackout curtains on all the windows. One evening they heard loud noises out side, they carefully peeked out the window and saw enemy troops coming up the street, they were entering every home, to pillage, and cause destruction. They had no way to protect themselves, and Alice was very frightened.

Alice knew here father was a righteous man, yet she was surprised by how calm he was, he simply said , "Don't be scared." He had them all kneel down and each offered a fervent prayer asking for protection. Her father a man of great faith prayed first , "Father in Heaven, please blind those soldiers. Make our house invisible so they won't see it."   After each had pleaded for safety from Heavenly Father they discreetly pulled back the blackout curtain and peered out into the night. The soldiers were still rampaging each house and were getting closer. Alice's family lived at the end of the street, and they saw the soldiers had not skipped one home on their block. To the great relief of the family, the enemy approached their house, but went right by the front gate and on to the next section of homes, the next street.

It was as though they didn't see their home. Alice goes on to say, "The next day I learned from a distraught friend that the soldiers had done terrible things in every house she knew of. When I told her that they had not come to our house, she was shocked. She said she had watched them go in our direction and that she knew of no homes in our sector that they had not entered. Our house was the only one the soldiers had left alone." Alice remembers this vividly from 65 years ago, and is so thankful to know that God hears our prayers. We are all trying to learn and understand faith , Alice's father felt calm and peace , he put his trust in Heavenly Father , doing all he could under these difficult circumstances. Their first defense was, faith, adding prayer, and trusting in the Lord. They were protected.

Chapter 5

EMOTIONS

RECOGNIZE - - RELEASE - - REPLACE

Many member, in drinking of the bitter cup that has come to them, wrongfully think that this cup passes by others.------------------"Having drunk the bitter cup, however, there comes a time when one must accept the situation as it is and reach upward and outward. President Harold B. Lee said, " Do not let self-pity or despair beckon you from the course you know is right."

(President James E. Faust; "A Second Birth"   1998 *Ensign* pg. 2)

Emotions, are they good or bad, can they help us or hurt us? - - well the answer is yes to both of them. Because of our feelings, emotions, we are able to experience things more deeply. We feel an emotion and it is also expressed in our physical body. Watch a baby cry, he is feeling frustration, or anguish, he expresses it in his tiny body, with his arms and legs flailing and is only interrupted briefly by his need to take a breath of air. Everyone within the sound of his wailing knows there is definitely something troubling the baby. Contrast this with listening to a small one laugh. It is delightful, such a cheerful, happy sound, it brightens our day and we cannot help but giggle. Whether the infant is playing peek-a-boo with mommy, or watching his brother make funny faces, it is expressed in the big smile, the happy countenance and again the arms and legs may be moving up and down, but this time it is because of joy, or delight.

God has given everyone the Light of Christ, which is the conscience of man.

"It is also "the light that quickeneth man's understanding" (D. & C. 88:6-13, 42) In this manner, **the light of Christ is related to man's conscience** and tells him right from wrong. (Moro. 7:12-19)   *Bible Dictionary, pg 725*

During our growing up years, we learn many technics for dealing with these emotions and yet some seem automatic, as if we came here to earth with them. Our emotions are felt in our physical body, they are expressed through our actions. Imagine you are at a basketball game, and your team is one point behind. This is the championship playoff. The tenseness is thick in the air, the cheerleaders are leading the supporters in chants , "You're a Winner - - You Can do It - Go team Go." The stadium is filled with spectators each cheering for their own team. Many people are standing, waving their arms, some even stomping. They each are excited for their team to win. There are only 5 seconds left in the game. A time out is called, each coach making last minute commands. The teams come back on the court, the referee throws the ball up and each of the team captains jump for the ball. As the ball descends, your team catches it and makes a long throw to their best shooter. He shoots, and the ball drops through the basket as the final buzzer is ringing. The stadium goes wild. The excitement in the air is electric. The team you have cheered for years finally won the State Championship.

You are jumping up and down, hugging your friends and giving high fives. You heart is racing because your team just won the championship. You have a grin on your face from ear to ear. You just expressed your great happiness through actions of your physical body.

Now take a look at the team that just lost and the people who wanted them to win. You don't have to ask which side they were cheering for.. Their shoulders may be slumped, they may be hugging their friends , but in a different way, to console, not to congratulate. Some may be angry, because they thought the referee, didn't make the calls right. There is a

79

sadness in their faces, their head is down. It is expressed in their actions. Some are wiping their eyes or even crying because their team lost.

In the cartoon "Peanuts" we see Lucy looking at Charlie Brown, he is standing with his head down and his shoulders slumped, he says, "This is my depressed stance." Then Charlie looks at her and says "When you're depressed, it makes a lot of difference how you stand." in the third frame he is standing up straight with his head up and says, "The worst thing you can do is straighten up and hold your head high because then you'll start to feel better." The final picture shows Charlie again with his head down, looking at the ground and his shoulders are again slumped - - "If you're going to get any joy out of being depressed you've got to stand like this." (From Anthony Robbins book; *Notes from a Friend*, pg 64, Anthony received permission from PEANUTS REPRINTED BY PERMISSION OF UFS. INC. 1960 United Feature Syndicate, Inc.)

Our physical actions affect our emotions, and vise versa, when we are feeling sad or depressed we look down, at our feet, at the ground, it is hard to find any joy in life, our head is down and shoulders slumped. We show in our physical body how we feel emotionally, or to say it another way, our physical body mirrors our emotions.

The Lord understands all of this perfectly. The prophet Alma spent much time and energy teaching the word of God in the city of Ammonihah. He did not just go out on the last day of the month to get his visiting or home teaching assignment done. He desired with all his heart for the people of this city to have the word of God

Alma 8:10, He labored much in the spirit, wrestling with God in mighty prayer, that he would pour out his Spirit upon the people who were in the city; that he would also grant that he might baptize them unto repentance. Alma 8:15 ; "Lift up thy head and rejoice."

Now take this same scenario and do a replay with no show of

80

physical emotions. Well your team play as good, putting their heart and soul into the game. If you feel excited mentally, you force yourself to not cheer, or wave your arms, but you may be bursting inside

Thought, creates emotions, and this is energy either positive or negative. Other people can feel it, see it, sense it. Look at a young couple in love, they smile at each other, they are holding hands , they look at each other and seem to have a light in their eyes, they almost have an inner glow, the positive vibrations just flow. Check out another couple that just had an argument. A totally different story, the emotions and energy are negative, it is uncomfortable being around them, no one has to tell you a thing, you just know, you feel the negative vibes.

Robert T. Kiyosake, from his book, Rich Dad - Poor Dad
Explained it this way, "Emotions are what make us human. Make us real. The word emotion stands for Energy in motion.. Be truthful about your emotions, and use your mind and your emotions in your favor."

Mark Twain once remarked that he had been through some terrible things in life - "SOME OF WHICH ACTUALLY HAPPENED."

Fit and Healthy.

Word of Wisdom -- D.&C. 89, D.& C. 88:123,124 "Arise early retire early, that your minds and bodies may be invigorated."

Here is a great key to what we should be looking for. Sustained energy,

D. & C. 59: 18 & 19 "Yea, all things which come of the earth, in the season thereof, are made for the benefit and use of man, both to please the eye and to gladden the heart;

"Yea, for food and for raiment, for taste and for smell, to strengthen the body and to enliven the soul."

Verse 20, " And it pleaseth God that he hath given all these things unto man, for unto this end were they made to be used, with judgment , not to excess, neither by extortion."

God created all these things, to strengthen the body and to enliven the soul. Does that give us a clue and ideas of what we should eat.

If we could all live in the Garden of Eden, I'm sure we would all be trim and fit and have an abundance of energy. There would be no artificial any thing. Everything in it's pure and natural state, full of vitamins and minerals   and anything the body needed. You just pick what you want, fresh from the tree or plant and within minutes you enjoy it's benefits. I am sure the taste would be absolutely wonderful.

What foods will give us sustained , long lasting energy. Do energy drinks fit and give us sustained energy??   It depends on how we choose them. Their lists of ingredients is a clue.

Gail Jackson, in the June 2007 issue of Desert Saints Magazine, came up with some things for us to think about. Gail says, " In the last few years new types of strong drinks have made their appearance and are being marketed in designs to delude us and our children."

"Today's energy drinks are filled with stimulants - - -massive amounts of caffeine, plus taurine, and guarana, both unregulated stimulants that intensifies caffeine's affect." Caffeine is not a flavoring agent. Its sole purpose is to stimulate and addict. Caffeine is a drug. When it is consumed in high amounts, it manipulates the pleasure center of the brain in a similar way that alcohol, tobacco, and illicit drugs do."

Our bodies were given to us from God, He refers to them as

temples. We only get one, we can't abuse it and then like a car go to the dealership and purchase a new one. There are doctors and skilled professionals that can help us if we break a bone or are in an accident and lose an arm or leg. They can help us with an artificial limb, but in the best cases, it does not work as well as the original .

There are so many things to learn in this life and taking care of our physical body is a high priority. We have our mind to govern our body. Our spirit is to be in charge.

Part of having your own sunshine, is having the energy and strength, to be able to CARRY, the Sunshine. The wrong kind of energy drinks may artificially accomplish the purpose for a time, and perhaps if you are driving on a long trip, it is much better to stay awake than have an accident, these are choices we have to make. It is difficult to accomplish much if you don't feel good. God has given guidelines from our living prophets, and the scriptures on how to keep our body healthy and strong.

Mental clarity, is so important , it is difficult to make correct decisions when our mind is groggy, or we are sleepy. The Lord made our bodies, and he certainly knows what is best to keep our bodies running the most efficient. He is the manufacture , he knows what we need. If you have a new car, you are going to do everything possible to keep it in good condition, after all you paid, or are still paying a lot of money to have such a shinny new vehicle. You probably would like it to last for many years. Generally you need to change the oil every 2,000 miles , Have a tune up, rotate the tires, and drive sensible, you definitely don't want an accident. Or even a small tiny scratch or even a little fender bender. The owners manual has a whole list of things that tells you how to keep your vehicle in the best condition.

We are to use wisdom in the foods we eat. Each person is different, and their body may not be able to handle wheat, or corn, peanuts, or any other of a number of things. They may have allergies that prevent them

83

from eating certain foods. What works for one person may not benefit another, yet here are some ideas that you might want to consider.

Our son Paul has his physical body in great shape.   He works out about 5 days a week at the gym. Which builds his muscles and also strengthens his heart. He alternates the workout so he can work each set of muscles, plus does an aerobic on alternate days to get his heart rate up.

I asked him what he has for his meals. He tries to eat every 2 or 3 hours, lean protein, with some veggies, or fruit, and perhaps some whole grain. He is very consistent. Yet occasionally for a special dinner or date., or birthday he will eat whatever he wants .

What we are looking for is what foods will give you the longest, most sustained energy, that is healthy for you. Again, if we were in the Garden of Eden anything we ate would be live and vibrant, full of live enzymes, and it would probably be raw. The soil would not be depleted of nutrients, the plants would grow properly. There would be no chemical fertilizers. With the sun, and the soil and the water it would grow perfectly. Since none of us are living in Eden now, we look for the best solution with what is available to us.

Having our own organic garden will provide much, but not everyone is in a situation to do this. Our son Seth who lives in Portland with his wife Gayle, love to plant and get things growing. In their Condo , they had a little tiny space of a yard, it is surprising the things they could grow there, tomatoes, peppers, lettuce, herbs. We had a fresh salad mainly from their garden, it was yummy.

There are hundreds of different eating plans, or some people would call them diets. I prefer to call it eating healthy for Life. It is a way of eating that is best for you, to help you be at the weight you like, with your clothes fitting more like you want. With the foods you eat helping provide you with optimum health, strength, and energy.

One major factor is portion size.. I was very impressed with my sister, Sandra, I could tell that she had lost or dis-guarded about 20 pounds, since I had last visited with her. What was her secret , what did she do differently. I noticed that she measured her servings , 1/2 cup vegies , 1 slice of bread , how much lean meat, or protein. I was impressed. She set the food in front of her, enjoyed each bite, and that is all she ate . She was finished. Wow, she certainly controlled her portion sizes.

Her husband Louis brought up an idea that he had learned from his dad. His father was getting up in years and his health was not as good as it used to be so he wasn't as active as he had been in years past doing lots of farm work. He said "Louis, to keep from gaining a lot of weight as you get older, take the amount of food you would normally eat, put it on your plate, then take half of it and move it to the side, and only eat half of what you used to. You'll be surprised that this amount will satisfy you. Louis is evidently doing this, he hasn't gained a lot of weight.

I read an article in Woman's World several years ago, {Nov. 29, 05} this woman in her 30's was over 100 lbs beyond her desired weight. She had tried many diets, would lose weight and be real pleased, but in a short time she would gain the weight back plus more. It was very, very discouraging for her.

One morning when she was very hungry, and looking for something quick to grab, she found the chicken fingers that were left over from the night before. She ate them plus some broccoli and was surprised at how satisfied she was, she skipped the junk food   She had some more for lunch and again was amazed at the energy she had and how she felt. That evening she was barely hungry, and a bowl of cereal was plenty. She decided to flip - flop her meals. Instead of eating junk food for breakfast, and the protein in the evening, she turned everything around. She started her day with protein - veggie's and some carbs . In the evening she would have cold cereal, with milk, or spaghetti with fat free cheese. She was

85

satisfied with less. She was amazed at how having lean protein made such difference in her extreme hunger.

Do you eat breakfast?? Many people who want to lose weight, start the day by saying I'll skip breakfast, then I will only eat a little the rest of the day, and the pounds will start to come off. This sounds good in theory, but our bodies need fuel to run on and we get hungry. Usually what happens when we try this by lunch time we are very hungry, so if we are working out of the home, we may grab a doughnut, or candy bar or a soft drink.

Then in a couple of hours we are hungry again, and get another quick fix of sugar and carbs. We get home in the evening, we haven't eaten much or think we have eaten hardly anything so we really enjoy dinner There was an interesting study that had volunteers eat only one meal a day. They each received   one meal a day which had 2,000 calories. They had half of the people eat their meal at breakfast, the other in the evening for dinner. The results were surprising. The ones who ate their food in the evening, gained weight. Those who ate their food in the morning lost weight. Same amount of calories, yet the difference was the time of day they ate. Why would that make such a difference. By eating the meal in the morning they still had 10 to 14 hours ahead of them, where they would be active, doing things which needed those calories for fuel - work - - errands - - house work -- - etc. They would be doing something.
On the other hand eating the 2,000 calorie meal in the evening, you would have only 3 to 4 or 5 hours that you would be active, and then probably much less than during the day. They would probably spent part of the time relaxing, unwinding , reading or watching T.V. Not much physical activity.

My husband and I like to go to buffets and here in Las Vegas, there are plenty. We only go once a week, or less. I enjoy whatever I want to eat, and I'm sure I eat too much , but I figure I will really enjoy this food. And I do. We used to go in the evening, and of course try all of the tempting, array, and variety. Then to top it off , by trying many of the desserts.

We would arrive home, very full. Did we do much when we got home - - of course not, and within a couple of hours we would have gone to bed. I always weigh myself every morning. The scales we have are the same you would see in a Doctors office. It is easy to tell if you are up or down in your weight, it is very accurate. You can even get it to a 1/4th of a pound that way I know exactly where I am at, and I knew I would have gained 2 or 3 pounds. And sure enough it was very true.

I thought maybe I'll try a different approach. Why not enjoy the buffet in the morning. I decided to experimented with the one meal a day, (only on the day we go to the buffet). I ate whatever I wanted, I'm sure it was well over 2,000 calories , they do have a big variety of foods, omelets, hash browns, bacon, yogurt, cereal, doughnuts and sweet rolls at breakfast buffets, plus much more. The breakfast buffet was the only meal I ate that day. The moment of truth came the next morning when I weighed my self, I was very pleased, I had not gained an ounce. So for me it worked as they said it did on the test group. I'm sure if I kept my calories to 2000, instead of much more I would have lost weight.

Is this wise and using wisdom?? Of course not. But it sure tasted good.

There is a saying, eat breakfast like a king, lunch like a prince and dinner like a pauper   It is good advice.

For years I looked for an eating plan that would work for me. One that would give me sustained energy and help me look more trim and fit. One that I could live with the rest of my life. Although I have rarely been on a diet, I would try new approaches.

One that I tried was very low fat. Hum.............. well I can eat what I want just as long as my fat intake is no more than 20% of the total calories. I ate healthy low treats like   whole grain fig newtons, plus other healthy food. I would check the package and see the percentage of   fat to the calories. I ate fruit, vegetables , whole grains. Yet I was surprised   I was not discarding pounds.   My tummy was bigger than I wanted. When I get extra pounds it goes to my tummy , and waist. Some people it goes to their hips.

We took a trip to see our son and daughter in law in Taiwan . We had not see them for several years. I had to laugh when my daughter in law said. "Mom you really do like to eat don't you."

Another friend of mine whose body type is the same as mine had one of her grandchildren pat her tummy, and say -- "Grandma, is there a baby in your tummy?"

I faithfully kept a record of what I ate, and did not exceed the fat percentages and would eat between 2000 - and 3000 calories a day. It did not work for me.

Each person is different, find what works for you. I have seen plans that call for 1/2 cup of oatmeal, fat free milk for breakfast , then a green salad with chicken breast, with fat free dressing for lunch. Veggies, and Salmon with 3/4 cup of pasta for dinner. I could not live on an eating plan like that for the rest of my life. I needed something with foods I like. I can't stand fat free milk, and my body doesn't digest it well. I would be very, very hungry on a plan that has only about 1,200 calories a day. The foods sounded good, but there was very little fat.

Your body needs fat to help it function properly.

There are some creative ideas that people use to motivate themselves to discard extra pounds. An interesting story is from "Chicken Soup for the Soul Shaping the New You." Jack Canfield & Mark Victor

Hansen are the co authors of the book. This story "A Bag of   Potatoes" by April Knight.

"I squinted at the woman in the photo taken at my aunt's birthday party. "Who is that fat lady sitting next to uncle John?" I asked. My aunt hesitated and then answered, "It's you."

April, was shocked, she had been in denial , when her clothes were too tight she would just buy a larger size. She used to be a size 10 but over the last 2 years she had gained 50 pounds, that is 25 lbs. a year , She had gone to her doctor hoping he would give her a medical reason for her weight gain since diabetes and heart trouble ran in her family. No such luck, he was very blunt and said,
"You're two pounds away from being obese because you eat too much and you don't do any exercise. Lose weight or die," he said.

Now there was no more excuses for April, she had justified herself because there had been a divorce, and her children were grown and on their own.. There was no one but herself at home , no husband to try and look nice for, she had no social life, no friend to exercise or to diet with.
All of her reasons for being fat, medical, social, being alone were dissolved, she had to really look at herself. She didn't like what she had become, and she finally realized that she had to take care of herself. She could not blame her situation in life on other things. She decided even if her social life was not as she wanted, it would be worth it to take care of herself. So she could feel good about her life.

With this new idea in her mind while shopping at the grocery store she saw a 10 pound bag of potatoes , she thought, "this is how I feel, heavy & lumpy, dull and uninteresting."

April bought the bag of potatoes, she imagined it was 10 lbs. of fat, ugly, heavy, and bulky. Immediately she had a plan, she was going to get rid of extra weight. The potatoes became her motivation - she carried them up the stairs, they were awkward and she imagined it was her own fat. Then she carried them down the stairs. Even when she was watching T. V. she had the bulky bag of potatoes on her lap.

She changed her eating habits to 4 small meals a day, and had nothing but fruit & water after the sun went down. When she lost her first pound April took out a potato, and as more pounds came off, the bag of potatoes got smaller. Ten pounds gone! April didn't stop there she bought another bag, and again packed them up and down the stairs. She was thrilled when she had lost 31 pounds.

People began to notice that she was losing weight and asked how she did it. She told them it was her potato diet. But no she never ate the potatoes. April has more energy, she walks to the library , she has joined a book discussion group an made new friends. She knows the next time she sees herself in a photo, it will be the real April and she will be proud of who she has become.

To have control over our emotions, we must have control over our thoughts. What do we think about, what do we say when we talk to ourselves. Do we build ourselves up or mentally criticize all the things we haven't accomplished. Do we judge ourselves against our neighbor because they have a better car, home, kids accomplish more. What is the mental picture in our minds.

Michelle Glauser, March 2011 *New Era* The Girl with the Beautiful Smile explains what happened to her. Michelle had been practicing for months for a competition in which students are judged on playing a memorized piece , how well they sound, expression, interpretation , etc. Also they would be judged on their verbal presentation of a composer. Even though Michelle's hands shook as she played her piece she was very relieved when it was over. Only one more thing left in the contest, to give her report.

She found the area and waited in line. But there were two doors. Michelle said, "Curiously, I looked in the door on the left. A friendly teacher encouraged students as they nervously entered and became acquainted. She obviously wanted to put them at ease."   Michelle continues, "Then I looked in the room on the right. There was another piano teacher, an older one, but she had a stern look that made my hands turn cold. The more I saw her interact with the students, the more scared I felt. All I could think was, "I hope I get the first judge." As Michelle waited, her fears increased, she hoped she would get the first judge, but just as it was about her turn to go in, another student on the right saw the door open and she walked into the room with the friendly, positive person. She panicked , her heart was racing she knew she would not have a chance with the negative teacher.

Then an idea came to her mind. "Just put on your biggest smile." Michelle continues, "I walked in with a bounce in my step and the biggest smile I'd ever shown. Like they say, by acting happy, you feel happy." Michelle was acting, she smiled at the judge often, she spoke in a loud clear voice, she even began to feel confident. By the end of her report she again smiled and thanked the judge for her time. Michelle left feeling very good about her report the judge. Several months later her piano teacher was going over the comments of the judges, and the last comment was, "Michelle, the girl with the beautiful smile." This experience changed her life. Michelle changed her thoughts which changed her attitude and the physical act of smiling worked wonders. Now she faces challenges with, a new look, instead of being unwilling, she has decided to make it fulfillling and enjoyable.

We need to recognize our negative thinking and then replace the old thoughts with new positive thoughts. The Savior gives an example of this in **_Luke 11: 24-26._** "When the unclean spirit is gone out of a man, he walketh through dry places, seeking rest; and finding none, he saith, I will return unto my house whence I came out. And when he cometh, he findeth it swept and garnished. Then goeth he, and taketh to him seven other spirits more wicked than himself; and they enter in, and dwell there; and the last state of that man is worse than the first."

LUKE 11:24-26 unclean spirit left, and came back with more.

The "Wizard of Oz" is a classic. Dorothy and her dog Toto are caught up in a tornado in Kansas, and disappear from her Uncle and Aunts home. During her journey she meets many strange characters, the tin man (without a heart)   The cowardly lion who is almost frightened by his shadow, and two witches, the good witch from the east and the wicked witch from the west. It is a story about her trying to make it back to Kansas. Plus when she finally meets the Wizard of Oz   who is suppose to have magical powers and she hopes he will find a way she can go home.

Each of us may at times feel something like each of these characters. Let me explain an experience I had; Prolapse as a Senior Citizen. My hormones changed. My whole body changed. My internal organs began to droop and as they drooped my whole body suffered. Of course it was a physical crisis that even threatened my life, but more than that it was an emotional earthquake that threatened my very soul. What had I done to deserve this? Nothing..... well, no I had delivered ten babies and my body was simply worn out.

I also looked for a "wizard" that would allow me to return to my former self. The wizard I chose was not a true wizard. Even though he did his best by implanting a new mesh that was supposed to hold my internal organs in place. It did not work and for the next eight years my life was torn by a whole series of operations to correct the damage that the mesh caused as it migrated into many critical areas of my body. I had it cut out of my vagina, I had it cut out of my colon, I had two surgeries to get it cut out of my bladder. For every surgery I must have had two or three major tests that also upset my life. It was a devastating 8years. I never did find my wizard. My salvation was the support of my husband and my recognition of the absolute necessity of learning and applying the

92

principles of Carry Your Own Sunshine.

Chapter 6

FORGIVENESS

_____

"It is reported that President Brigham Young once said that he who takes offense when no offense was intended is a fool and he who takes offense when offense was intended is usually a fool. It was then explained that there are two courses of action to follow when one is bitten by a

rattlesnake. One may, in anger, fear, or vengefulness, pursue the creature and kill it. Or he may make full haste to get the venom out of his system. If we pursue the latter course we will likely survive but if we attempt to follow the former, we may not be around long enough to finish it."
(Brigham Young, *Conference Report, Oct. 1973, pp. 15-16: Ensign* Jan 1974, pp. 20-21)   From D.& C. Student Manuel

FORGIVE OTHERS------WHY???
(They did the wrong, not I)

One of the most difficult things to learn in this life is how to forgive. If in the pre-existence everyone was kind to us, and everyone loving, there would be no need to forgive. No one would be offended or hurt by others. Yet we are here to learn and develop the qualities of Jesus and Heavenly Father. How could we know if we really knew how to swim, unless we were in deep water. In theory we may have understood forgiveness, but not in practice.

"Be Ye therefore perfect, even as your Father which is in Heaven is perfect."   There was no one more forgiving than our Savior. "Father forgive them for they know not what they do."

The wondrous atonement that Jesus suffered was not only for the whole world, but for you and I, and even for the person who so terribly offended and hurt you. Wait, that can't be fair, they sinned , I did not!! God is fair and just and merciful, there ARE conditions for the sinner to be forgiven.

In D.&.C. Section 18, verse 11
"For, behold, the Lord your Redeemer suffered death in the flesh; wherefore he suffered the pain of all men, that all men might repent and come unto him."

So, there are conditions for the sinner------REPENTANCE!!

94

I can't forgive. The things they did to me were so terrible and wrong. Why should I forgive? The answers are in the scriptures. The Lord has told us the consequences of not forgiving.

"My disciples, in days of old, sought occasion against one another and forgave not one another in their hearts; and for this evil they were afflicted and sorely chastened.

"Wherefore, I say unto you, that ye ought to forgive one another; for he that forgiveth not his brother his trespasses standeth condemned before the Lord; for there remaineth in him the greater sin.

"I, the Lord, will forgive whom I will forgive, but of you it is required to forgive all men.
And ye ought to say in your hearts----let God judge between me and thee, and reward thee according to thy deeds." (D.& C. 64:9-11)
In the Book, "Love is Letting Go of Fear," by Gerald G. Jampolsky, M.D. page 35, Gerald explains, " Inner peace can be reached only when we practice forgiveness. Forgiveness is the letting go of the past. - - - - Through this process of selective forgetting, we become free to embrace a present without the need to reenact our past."

President Boyd K. Packer, in the *Conference Ensign*, May 2011, page 32. Tells the poignant story of a man who was a patriarch, and his extreme trial as a young married man.
His sweet wife was expecting their first child , and since this happened many years ago, there was only one doctor for the town and surrounding countryside. He made house calls and in his endeavors to help the sick was often run ragged, quickly moving from one area to another in his efforts to administer relief.   As the young mother went into labor there began to be complications and the Doctor was needed immediately. Locating the Dr. was difficult, but finally he was on his way. When he arrived he acted quickly and soon a new baby was welcomed into this couples home.

Everything seemed to be fine, however a few days later his lovely wife died of an infection that unknowingly was carried from another patient the Dr. was treating that very day. This young man was left with a new baby to care for and the heartache of his wife being gone. He became, angry, he could think of nothing else but getting even with the Doctor. Getting revenge, finding a way to have him suffer as much as he was. This was his constant focus, the anger the bitterness building day by day. "One night a knock came at his door. A little girl said simply, "Daddy wants you to come over. He wants to talk to you."

"Daddy" was the stake president. The counsel from that wise leader was simply "John, leave it alone. Nothing you do about it will bring her back. Anything you do will make it worse. John, leave it alone."

This was extremely difficult for the him, it seemed so unfair. It was unfair. His wife was gone , she would not be at his side to help raise their child. Why should he forgive? The Doctor should have to suffer as much as he was. Finally, not understanding he decided to be obedient and follow the Stake President's counsel.

"He said, I was an old man before I understood and could finally see a poor country doctor---overworked, underpaid, run ragged from patient to patient, with little medicine, no hospital, few instruments, struggling to save lives, and succeeding for the most part. He had come in a moment of crisis, when two lives hung in the balance, and had acted without delay.. I finally understood!"   He said, "I would have ruined my life and the lives of others."

He goes on to explain that after he finally understood , he many times prayed to Heavenly Father thanking him for a wise Stake President , who's simple counsel was "John, leave it alone."

President Packer gives a great analogy of someone who won't forgive and how it impacts their life. "That attitude is somewhat like a man being hit by a club. Offended, he takes up a club and beats himself over the head with it all the days of his life. How foolish! How Sad! That kind of revenge is self-inflicting. If you have been offended, forgive, forget, it and leave it alone."

D. & C. 58:42,43 , " Behold, he who has repented of his sins, the same is forgiven, and I, the Lord, remember them no more."   Think of how the Lord responded to Saul - - Paul, thou are a chosen vessel, Saul was responsible for Christians to be put in prison and to be killed   he held the coats when Steven was stoned. Yet the Lord did not keep bringing up his past sins. The Saints of that day had a difficult time even comprehending Saul had changed

The Lord is very clear, not forgiving one another is EVIL, and because of an unforgiving heart they were afflicted and sorely chastened.

Picture yourself on judgement day standing before the Lord. You have lead a good life, you attend your meetings, you do 100% of your home or visiting teaching, you have a temple recommend, yet you still have great anger and bitterness in your heart for a person who has done you great wrong.. What will be your thoughts and actions before the Lord. Will you say, Lord I am justified in not forgiving- - - - you can see what this person did to me. Surely you do not expect me to forgive them.

The Lord may say, "But if ye forgive not men their trespasses, neither will your Father for give your trespasses. (Matthew 6:15)

-- "for there remaineth in him the greater sin.."

The Lord makes it very clear, "I the Lord, will forgive whom I will forgive, BUT OF YOU IT IS REQUIRED TO FORGIVE ALL MEN. (Emphasis added)

How can not forgiving, be the greater sin? Steve F. Gilliland in an article in the August 2004 *Ensign*, entitled "Forgiveness Our Challenge and Our Blessing" page 46 gives a beautiful answer to this question..

"Sin is anything we permit into our lives that will destroy us spiritually. When we poison ourselves with vengeful feelings, with hate; we distance ourselves from the influence of the Spirit of the Lord. Not only that, but---we attempt to assume one of God's roles---that of determining who is worthy of "

No if's- - - and's - - - or - - -but's, we are to forgive even till 7 times 70. That is 490 times, just for one person who has hurt us. That is a lot.

How do we forgive? The Lord tells us how, "And ye ought to say in your hearts---let God judge between me and thee and reward thee according to they deeds."

But Lord, you don't understand what they did, or how deeply it has hurt me, my life and my loved ones. You're asking too much------I can't forgive!!

If we say we can't forgive because someone has deeply hurt us, and there are a multitude of ways we have been hurt, mentally, physically, emotionally, financially, to name a few; we are turning away from the very thing that will help us to heal.

There is an excellent example in the " written by Jane Mcbride Choate, "Pebble of Forgiveness "*Friend*, Feb. 2003, pg.42-44,   {Based on a true story).

Levi worked hard to earn money for his very own bicycle. He took good care of it and carefully put it away on a side wall in the garage. Jason his older brother, had just gotten his drivers license. While parking the car in the garage he hit Levi's bike and crumpled the fender.

Jason apologized several times, but Levi refused to listen. He was

98

angry with his brother. He felt Jason was not sorry for what he had done. Several days later in Primary sharing time Sister McClure passed a cup around the room and asked each child to take a small pebble from the cup.

"Put a pebble into your shoe," she said. "Now try walking in place."

The small stone felt very uncomfortable. It grew more irritating when they walked around the room. In fact it seemed almost as if it grew. It felt bigger and was beginning to hurt. After several minutes Sister McClure had the children remove the pebble from their shoe.

Then she explained, "Those little pebbles are like the feelings we have when we don't forgive someone who has offended us. They can start out small but then feel bigger and bigger."

"What if the person who did something to hurt us isn't really sorry?" Levi wanted to know.

"Sometimes we need to forgive, even when the other person doesn't apologize or repent," Sister McClure responded.

Later that day Levi told his parents about the pebble in his shoe.

"How did your foot feel by the time you took the pebble out?" His dad asked.

"My foot was a little sore," Levi admitted. "Sister McClure compared walking around with a pebble in your shoe to carrying a grudge and refusing to forgive someone who offended you."

Before he went to bed, Levi knocked on Jason"s door. "I'm sorry I've been such a jerk," he said when Jason opened the door. "I know you didn't mean to run over my bike."

"Hey, I'm the one who's sorry." Jason pulled Levi into a bear hug and lifted him off the floor. "What do you say we work on the bike together tomorrow after school?"

"Great!" Levi said, and as he went to his room, he thought, "I really do feel great!"

The Lord has commanded us to forgive. President Faust gently reminded us of this. "We encourage Church members to forgive those who may have wronged them." (Ensign, July 2002, 'A Priceless Heritage,' pg. 6

Elder Jeffrey R. Holland stated in Conference Oct. 1996, "We don't want God to remember our sins, so there is something fundamentally wrong in our relentlessly trying to remember those of others."

"When we have been hurt, undoubtedly God takes into account what wrongs were done to us and what provocations there are for our resentments, but clearly the more Provocation there is and the more excuse we can find for our hurt, all the more reason for us to forgive and be delivered from the destructive hell of such poisonous venom and anger." (Adapted from George Macdonald) It is one of those ironies of godhood that in order to find peace, the offended as well as the offender must engage the principles of forgiveness." Jeffrey R. Holland "The Peaceable Things of the Kingdom", *Ensign*, November 1996 Pg. 83,

In General Conference, Oct. 1973-----(Ensign, Jan. 1974, pg. 20-21) Elder Marion D. Hanks said,

"Someone has written: -----the withholding of love is the negation of the spirit of Christ, the proof that we never knew him, that for us he lived in vain. It means that he suggested nothing in all our thoughts, that we were not once near enough to him to be seized with the spell of his compassion for the world."

Refusing to forgive means we don't understand or accept the ATONEMENT OF OUR SAVIOR JESUS CHRIST.

It is difficult to forgive. It is much easier to get angry, and then work to get even, to try and inflict as much pain on the sinner as they inflicted on us. There is a false sense of power when someone is angry. A great analogy was given by Brigham Young,

"It is reported that President Brigham Young once said that he who takes offense when no offense was intended is a fool, and he who takes offense when offense was intended is usually a fool. It was then explained that there are two courses of action to follow when one is bitten by a rattlesnake. One may, in anger, fear, or vengefulness, pursue the creature and kill it. Or he may make full haste to get the venom out of his system. If we pursue the latter course we will likely survive, but if we attempt to follow the former, we may not be around long enough to finish it."
(Marion D. Hanks , "Even as Christ Forgave, "*New Era*, June 1974, Pg. 4-5)

Judge not, that ye be not judged. For with what judgment ye judge, ye shall be judged: And with what measure ye mete, it shall be measured to you again. Matt. 7:1-2

In his book "*The Miracle of Forgiveness*" pages 267-268 , President Spencer W. Kimball   say's;

"The Lord will judge with the same measurements meted out by us. If we are harsh, we should not expect other than harshness. If we are merciful with those who injure us, he will be merciful with us in our errors. If we are unforgiving, he will leave us weltering in our own sins."

"The Lord can judge men by their thoughts as well as by what they say and do, for he knows even the intents of their hearts; but this is not true of humans. We hear what people say, we see what they do, but being unable to discern what they think or intend, we often judge wrongfully if we try to fathom the meaning and motives behind their actions and place on them our own interpretation."

Why should we forgive? There are many reasons. First and most important, because Heavenly Father commanded us to, and our Savior showed the perfect example.

What if the things said about you are completely untrue, and you are devastated because it is from one you love and respect. How could they say such a thing and believe it.

In reading in the Book of Mormon we have a true life situation where this happened. In Alma chapters 60 and 61 Moroni (Who is the chief captain of the Nephite army) writes a scathing letter to Pahoran. Pahoran, is the chief Judge and the governor over the land and is in the city of Zarahemla.

Moroni is also directing his words to "all those who have been chosen by this people to govern and manage the affairs of this war.

The letter doesn't start out very positive.
verse 2 - - - "For behold, I have somewhat to say unto them by the way of condemnation; for behold, ye yourselves know that ye have been appointed to gather together men and arm them with swords, and with cimeters, and all manner of weapons of war of every kind, and send forth against the Lamanites, in whatsoever parts they should come into our land."

Moroni then proceeds to tell Pahoran all of the suffering they have experienced because of their great neglect.

V. 3 "---yea, even hunger, thirst, and fatigue, and all manner of afflictions of every kind."

If all of this didn't make Pahoran feel terrible, the next statement surely would.

V. 4 " But behold, were this all we had suffered we would not murmur nor complain.

V. 5. "But behold, great has been the slaughter among our people; yea thousands have fallen by the sword, while it might have otherwise been if you had rendered unto our armies sufficient strength and succor for them."

Moroni is very direct and doesn't spare words to make his point.

V. 6. "Can you think to sit upon your thrones in a state of thoughtless stupor, while your enemies are spreading the work of death around you? Yea, while they are murdering thousands of your brethren."

V. 18 "But why should I say much concerning this matter? For we know not but what ye yourselves are seeking for authority. We know not but what ye are also traitors to your country."

The words from Moroni to Pahoran are very direct and condemning. How would you feel if you were Pahoran and had just received such a letter, or epistle. Me a traitor???

Pahoran did not respond with anger or vengefulness, he did not try and get even.

After explaining their dire circumstances and the reason help was not given; in Alma 61:9 Pahoran states: "And now, in your epistle you have censured me, but It mattereth not; I am not angry, but do rejoice in the greatness of your heart."

What Christ like forgiveness Pahoran had, not for one instant did

103

he harbor any anger. He did not waste his time or energy being angry. He was falsely accused, slandered , yet he returned this anger with love.

Alma 61:14 "Therefore, my beloved brother, Moroni,"-----
He responded with love, and found positive things to say about this great leader.   He did not focus on anger, or hurt, or revenge, or the un-justice of the epistle. He was not stopped by negative feelings. He quenched the flames of the fire with love and kindness.

Contrast Pahoran's Christ like forgiveness with a young man I'll call Tom.. He was visiting our ward and since we knew him quite well he asked, who the man sitting across the isle was. When I gave Tom the man's name, I asked why he wanted to know. I was interested in his response, actually shocked by it.

"Well, I'm angry with him because he took 2 parking spaces instead of just one. He should know better. How can he be so inconsiderate and thoughtless. I'm going to talk to him right after church and let him know I'm angry with him."

Since we had known this young man for some time and we were friends, I said, "Tom , let it go!! It is not worth wasting your energy over this.

In analyzing this situation what were the results of Tom being angry?

First of all I doubt if Tom got much out of Sacrament meeting because he was focusing on how inconsiderate the other man was, and it was his duty to tell the man his faults and see that this wrong was made right.

Second because he was angry he began to let the spirit of darkness enter, and therefore the Spirit of the Lord would begin to withdraw, or be

104

restrained.

Evidently Tom stopped letting it bother him so much because later when I asked him about it, he said he saw the brother making sure the flowers were passed out for Mother's Day, so perhaps he had the flowers in his car, and was in a hurry to get them in the church.

By changing his thinking Tom was able to stop focusing on anger and begin to have a little understanding and compassion. Tom saw the injustice in black and white. That is wrong, this is right, but he didn't know the whole situation, and when he considered that this man may have been in a hurry to make sure the flowers were on time his heart softened.

Only the Lord knows the thoughts and intents of our heart.

.D&C 6:16, states, "Yea, I tell thee, that thou mayest know that there is none else save God that knowest thy thoughts and the intents of they heart."

How can we possibly judge another, we don't know their trials and their challenges and the difficulties they have had to face. In the Hymn, "Lord, I Would Follow Thee" pg. 220 This is explained beautifully. Verse 2. (Emphasis added)

"Who am I to judge another   When I walk imperfectly?
In the quiet heart is hidden   Sorrow that the eye can't see.
Who am I to judge another? Lord, I would follow thee.

Verse three explains what the Lord would have us do, how to help another.

"I would be my brothers's keeper; I would learn the healer's art.
To the wounded and the weary I would show a gentle heart.
I would be my brother's keeper   Lord, I would follow thee."

How can we help lift others when we are feel so inadequate ourselves. Verse four tells us where we will find strength.

"Savior, may I love my brother As I know thou lovest me,
Find in thee my strength, my beacon, For thy servant I would be.
Savior, may I love my brother Lord, I would follow thee."

An excellent example of forgiving is in the July 2001 *Ensign,* pages 67,68; written by Renee Roy Harding. "Could I Learn To Forgive?"

Renee tells how her mother was killed by a drunk driver when she was 21 years old, and the pain and heartache she had in trying to deal with the loss of her mother. It was even more difficult because Renee had quit attending church and started partying.

Just several hours before the accident she was yelling and angry at her mom.

Renee explains, "After Mom's death, as hard as I tried, I could find no peace, no solace, no answers in a world that had suddenly been turned upside down."

"I had been deliberately rebellious. Racked with shame and guilt, in anguish I prayed, begging for forgiveness. Soon I realized that Heavenly Father was the same kind of parent my mother had been; full of love and quick to hear my cries; even though I felt undeserving of both. I knew I could sob to my Heavenly Father the way I used to cry on my mom's shoulder."

"I met with my bishop many times in the months that followed. One night as I left the bishop's office, so happy to finally feel the heavy weight of my sins beginning to lift, I had a startling realization: Did I wish that the man who killed my mother would suffer and be punished forever

106

for his sins while I was forgiven for mine? And could I really expect to be forgiven if I was unwilling to forgive him?"

"It was clear to me that malice can slow or stop our eternal progression and separate us from the love of our Father in Heaven and the Savior. I knew more than ever that forgiveness was the key to the peace I so desperately craved.

She goes on to say, "Mr. Olsen and I were both so in need of mercy, forgiveness, and the peace of mind that comes from knowing we can be forgiven. Our very lives depended upon it."

Renee was able to forgive the man who accidentally killed her mother while driving intoxicated. She was able to personally tell him she forgave him.

How do you forgive when the wounds and the hurts are so deep. The physical scars may or may not be there, however the emotional scars are very deep.

President Gordon B. Hinckley said in the June 1991 Ensign Pages 2-5--
"If there be any who nurture in their hearts the poisonous brew of enmity toward another, I plead with you to ask the Lord for strength to forgive. This expression of desire will be of the very substance of your repentance. It may not be easy, and it may not come quickly. But if you will seek it with sincerity and cultivate it, it will come. . . .

"There is no peace in reflecting on the pain of old wounds. There is peace only in repentance and forgiveness. This is the sweet peace of the Christ, who said, 'blessed are the peacemakers; for they shall be called the children of God.'" (Matt. 5:9)

In order to forgive ask the great healer of all men, the Savior to help you. He understands , oh how he understands. As you sincerely pray to forgive, the Lord will take away the pain and the hurt in your soul and bring you peace. Such is a lifting of the burden.

President Spencer W. Kimball (1895-1985) , *The Miracle of Forgiveness* (1969), pg. 300

"It can be done. Man can conquer self. Man can overcome. Man can forgive all who have trespassed against him and go on to receive peace in this life and eternal life in the world to come."

Layne T. Derrick, [in the March 1980 "The New Era", pages 28,29, Missionary Focus, "Mirian"] gives an example of Christ like forgiveness. While serving as a missionary in Equador he met a young member of the church. Her name was Mirian, she was only 5 feet tall. The thing that was different about her was that she had no teeth, this was very unusual for someone her age.   Her father had died about a year earlier, and false rumors were spread about Mirian's mother.

She said, "One night I had had enough so I went out to defend my mother and what I knew was right. Several of those in the neighborhood decided to gang up on me and teach me a lesson, one I would never forget. They started to beat me, hitting me mostly in the face. This is how I lost all my teeth."

Mirian shared the gospel with many. Layne explaines, "I'll always remember the time we decided to talk with those who had harrassed Mirian so badly before. As if nothing had happened between them Mirian helped teach these families, several of who became converted to the gospel."

"I was transferred not long after this and shortly thereafter was shocked to learn that Mirian had died of complications following a ruptured appendix. Yet as sad as that was, she had accomplished a great mission. Because of her deep faith in the Lord and his powers to protect, Mirian had overcome her fear of her fellowmen and had helped to teach the gospel to those who had physically scarred her for life. Many of them now revere her name for forgiving them and bringing them the gospel of Jesus Christ."

An article in the Church News, November 4, 2001   states,

"One of human nature's ironies is that many want forgiveness for their own failings, sins or weaknesses, but seem to expect others to be held to a higher standard, to suffer long, to carry forever the weight of their sins.

Some hold in their memories the transgressions of others but fail to remember the cleansing power of repentance, that great gift proffered at the precious cost of the divine Atonement. At what point along life's time line does one "remember no more" Sins repented of by another And who are we to presume that more time must pass or more anguish must be endured before sin's stain fades into oblivion?"

Some people say, well I can forgive, but I will never forget. When the Lord say's I will remember them no more are we to do less.

President Spencer W. Kimball in his book "*The Miracle of Forgiveness*" page 299, clarifies it even more.

" If we have been wronged or injured, forgiveness means to blot it completely from our minds. To forgive and forget is an ageless counsel. "To be wronged or robbed," said the Chinese philosopher Confucius, "is nothing unless you continue to remember it."

This is a poem written by my son Seth Sinclair, December 1999 while he was on his mission in Paraguay.

FORGIVENESS IS THE KEY

Forgiveness is the Key I've missed for many sins I've had,
Not upon the receiving end, but of the giving hand.

For I've received forgiveness for many sins I've made.
At the times I've been forgiven I didn't cut the grade.

Those people who forgave me for so very many times,
I don't know how they did it, considering my crimes.

For I have Loved and lost, and I have learned to love.
I have seen the pain beneath and felt the joy above.

But through the trials of my life, the joys and the pains.
When someone does me wrong it seems the anger still
remains.

The throbbing in my heart, the hatred from within.
These people that have wronged me, I can not let them win.

The pain that they have caused me, the things that I have lost
The anger building up inside, is it worth the cost?

The cost of losing sleep, the cost of wasting time,
only thinking of the wrongs they did, and how terrible
their crimes.

These feelings kept me going, the hatred kept me strong.
The fear that they had caused me is not quite completely
gone.

At times when I'm alone at night, with that unfamiliar sound,

I see the flash backs of the pain they caused, and my heart
begins to pound.

Then fear enters in my mind, as if it's happening again.
The pictures running through my head and I relive their sin.

But I am so accustomed, I've felt this way for years.
I am a little scared to have a life without my tears.

I don't know how I'd make it, could I still be strong;
by forgiving and forgetting, these pains I've held so long?"

My father and Uncle both had dairy farms. They had one set of
horses that they shared. Their farms were about 1 quarter mile apart. Their
was a disagreement and hurt feelings. This may have even happened
before I was born, but even though nothing was said to me as I got older I
realized that my Father and Uncle never spoke to each other. I had no idea
why. This continued on them never speaking at family gatherings and etc,
till my father died. After the funeral my Uncle came up and said to my
mother I wish I had talked to your father before this. Well, I wish my
father had talked to my Uncle before he died. It is sad that the hurt and the
pride and the pain were carried for so many years. The one good thing was
they didn't carry their feud to us children. My Uncle's daughter & I spent
many afternoons playing and having fun. To this day we are good friends.

I'm glad this family situation didn't carry over for generations, as
did Lamen and Lemuel, feeling their brother Nephi robbed them and took
over ruling them. This incorrect tradition was carried on for hundred's of
years.

In April Conference 2002, President Thomas S. Monson talks
about forgiving, "Hidden Wedges", *Ensign* May 2002, pg19,20

"Some time ago I read the following Associated Press dispatch, which appeared in the newspaper. An elderly man disclosed at the funeral of his brother, with whom he had shared, from early manhood, a small, one-room cabin near Canisteo, New York, that following a quarrel, they had divided the room in half with a chalk line and neither had crossed the line or spoken a word to the other since that day---62 years before. What a powerful and destructive hidden wedge."

In the same article President Monson says, "The spirit must be freed from tethers so strong and feelings never put to rest, so that the lift of life may give buoyancy to the soul. In many families, there are hurt feelings and a reluctance to forgive. It doesn't really matter what the issue was. It cannot and should not be left to injure. Blame keeps wounds open. Only forgiveness heals. George Herbert, an early 17th -century poet, wrote these lines: He that cannot forgive others breaks the bridge over which he himself must pass if he would ever reach heaven, for everyone has need of forgiveness."

How do you forgive?

1. First of all turn to the Lord, with mighty prayer. Tell the Lord how you really feel, if you are angry, upset, mad, hurt. The mental anguish, and pain. How the sinner has caused you so much hurt and emotional trauma. How it has affected you life and the lives of those you love. These feelings have been festering inside your mind. They are the last thing you think of before you go to bed and the first thought in the morning. At times even your dreams wake you with bad memories. Be completely open and honest with the Lord. You can tell Him anything and everything. He already knows your thoughts and why you feel as you do. As you shed tears of hurt and anguish He is there with compassion, love and understanding. He will listen, He does listen , The Lord is the best listener I have ever known.

The hymn "Where Can I turn for Peace?" page 129 of our hymn book explains clearly who we can turn to.

112

Where can I turn for peace? Where is my solace
When other sources cease to make me whole?
When with a wounded heart, anger or malice
I draw myself apart, Searching my soul?

Where, when my aching grows, Where, when I languish,
Where, in my need to know, where can I run?
Where is the quiet hand to calm my anguish?
Who, who can understand? He, only One.

He answers privately, Reaches my reaching
In my Gethsemane, Savior and Friend.
Gentle the peace he finds for my beseeching.
Constant he is and kind, Love without end.

He will guide and direct and help change your heart. By forgiving
we can again experience, peace and joy and happiness in our life.

In the "Church News" June 12, 1983   page 15 "Miracle awaits
forgivers" Ilene Condie explains her struggle to forgive, and then the
happiness she felt by forgiving.

"During my desperate struggle to forgive someone who had deeply
hurt me, I received instructions from my bishop to finish reading President
Spencer W. Kimball's book, *The Miracle of Forgiveness.* In addition, he
told me to read the scriptures and pray. I was also impressed to make
amends with a neighbor with whom words had destroyed our friendship.

I'll never forget that Tuesday morning in my kitchen when I
actually experienced the miracle of forgiveness. The windows of heaven
were open and so much joy, happiness and laughter filled my soul, I could
not control them. I also felt my Heavenly Father's great love for me and

His forgiveness for the things I had done wrong. What a cleansing. I actually felt squeaky clean.

The misery we put ourselves through for not forgiving others is crazy when we could be gaining spiritual growth and happiness."

Why forgive? First the Lord commanded us to forgive. If we don't forgive we could be so carried away in our hurt and anger and bitterness, that our progression is slowed or stopped. Are we looking to the Savior if we haven't forgiven.

"Look unto me in every thought, doubt not fear not."
D.& C. 6:36

Give your hurts and sufferings to the Lord. If you can't forgive ask Him to help you. He will, He understands, He knows the burdens you are carrying. An article in the Ensign, April 2002 explains the burdens we carry by not forgiving.

The woman in the article was very lonely and depressed. She did not feel any love for her husband even though years before the Spirit had whispered that this was to be her companion. Her feelings were that he needed to change for things to get better.

"When my heart was finally broken, I conceded to Him that I was incapable of resolving this problem on my own. When I became willing to accept whatever the Lord would tell me, I became painfully aware that I was part of the problem and that for our marriage to continue, I needed to forgive."

She says that her husband committed no major sins , just the everyday challenge of two people sharing their lives.

"Now I faced the realization that my inability to forgive was the major roadblock to a successful marriage."

"Accepting this truth, I resolved I would do better. However, just telling myself that I wanted to forgive was not changing my feelings. Years of harbored resentment had created wounds that would not easily heal, so I struggled to let go of all my hurt and pain."

"Feeling powerless to change my feelings, I cried out in prayer, "Father, please help me forgive-----through the power of Jesus Christ, the Redeemer of this world."

"A feeling of peace swept through my body, and I felt renewed in every part of my being. In amazement, I thanked heavenly Father for the gift He had given me. My hurt was swept away, my pains were erased, and love beyond description filled my heart."   April, 2002 Ensign, "I cried out to my Father" name withheld.

Why forgive?   The blessed inner peace.

Change your focus, what are you thinking of , if you see a bad movie, would you see it again? Why replay the terrible deed in your mind. As the poem, "Forgiveness is the Key" says, why relive the deed, over and over again, the pain, the anguish, the hurt. Why let someone else's actions determine your attitude. Why feel miserable because of the actions of others.

Jan Bittner in the "Church News, 1 May 1999, page 15 shares how she eventually was able to completely forgive by controlling her thoughts.

"I had a bad marriage. I knew that it was important to forgive, so I fasted and prayed and studied the scriptures and, after some years, thought I had managed to forgive. Then, my ex-husband died and I was shocked to find I was glad. I had all that work to do again. I eventually felt that I had forgiven him. Then a good friend told me that it seemed to be out of

115

character for me to be so bitter. I was surprised.

What more could I do? I prayed about it, asking, this time, what I could do more. Eventually, the answer came. "Control your thoughts!" So I kept track of my thinking, and when I found myself being negative, I amended my thoughts to something positive. This, along with fasting and prayer, brought me the peace I had yearned for. This time, I really have forgiven."

Ann M. Madsen , at BYU Women's Conference 1997, talked about the difficulty of forgiving. She mentioned she was having a hard time forgiving someone who had passed on several years before. She explains that as she was sitting in Sacrament Meeting she felt this personal revelation from the Lord.

"Forgiveness is one of our tasks as we partake of the Sacrament. If we would be forgiven, we must ourselves forgive. To truely forgive, I must idently the hurt, the pain and then offer it as a willing sacrifice to God. It is in my heart that the mighty change can take place.

Chapter 7

TRIALS

Whatever Jesus lays HIS HANDS UPON LIVES. IF JESUS LAYS HIS HANDS UPON A MARRIAGE, IT LIVES. IF HE IS ALLOWED TO LAY HIS HANDS ON THE FAMILY, IT LIVES." President Howard W. Hunter , General Conference, 1979, *Church News*----29 December 2001

TRIALS (The refiners fire)

THE SILVERSMITH

Some time ago, a few ladies met to study the scriptures. While reading the third chapter of Malachi, they came upon a remarkable expression in the third verse; "And He shall sit as a refiner and purifier of silver." (Malachi 3:3)

One lady decided to visit a silversmith, and report to the others on what he said about the subject. She went accordingly, and without telling him the reason for her visit, begged the silversmith to tell her about the process of refining silver.

After he had fully described it to her, she asked, "Sir, do you sit while the work of refining is going on?"

"Oh, yes ma'am," replied the silversmith;   "I must sit and watch the furnace constantly, for, if the time necessary for refining is exceeded in the slightest degree, the silver will be injured."

The lady at once saw the beauty and comfort of the expression, **"He shall sit as a refiner and purifier of silver."**

God sees it necessary to put His children into the furnace; But His eye is steadily intent on the work of purifying, and His wisdom and love are both engaged in the best manner for us. Our trials do not come at random, and He will not let us be tested beyond what we can endure.

Before she left, the lady asked one final question, "How do you know when the process is complete?"

"That's quite simple," replied the silversmith. "When I can see my own image in the silver, the refining process is finished."   Author unknown

The purpose of trials is to refine us....

In Moroni 7:45-48 Charity is explained—"And charity suffereth long and is kind, and envieth not, and is not puffed up, seeketh not her own, is not easily provoked, thinketh no evil, and rejoiceth not in iniquity but rejoiceth in the truth, beareth all things, believeth all things hopeth all things, endureth all things."

From the above verse these two words jump out at me, suffereth long-----------endureth all things. The refining process is difficult and intense. There is a furnace and fire, the mental, emotional and physical pain at times are more than we think we can bare. That is why the silversmith sits and watches the furnace constantly. God is in charge. He knows all things. He knows the strengths and weaknesses we came to earth with. He suffered all things for us. He wants us to become like Him.

Verse 48 - - ------ - -- *that when he shall appear we shall be like him,* for we shall see him as he is; that we may have this hope; that we may be purified even as he is pure.

In Alma chapter 5 verse 14 - - - - Have ye received his image in your countenances? Have you experienced this mighty change in your hearts?"

And in verse 19 - - - - - -I say unto you can you look up, having the image of God engraven upon your countenances?

How do we become more like the Savior? We look to Him. We learn of Him. We study His life through the scriptures. As the Savior said in D.& C. 6:36, " Look unto me in every thought; doubt not, fear not." We put our faith and trust in the Savior.

Elder Bruce R. McConkie explained the testing of the Saints in mortality:

"The testing processes of mortality are for all men, saints and sinners alike. Sometimes the tests and trials of those who have received the gospel far exceed any imposed upon worldly people. - - - -------Saints in all ages have been commanded to lay all that they have upon the altar, sometimes even their very lives.

"As to the individual trials and problems that befall any of us, all we need say is that in the wisdom of Him who knows all things, and who does all things well, all of us are given the particular and specific tests that we need in our personal situations.--- - - - - - - -

"But come what may, anything that befalls us here in mortality is but for a small moment, and if we are true and faithful God will eventually exalt us on high.   All our losses and sufferings will be made up to us in the resurrections." (Bruce R. McConkie ,*Conference Report, Oct. 1976 pp. 158-160 or Ensign,* Nov. 1976, pp. 106, 108.)

President Brigham Young said, "If the Saints could realize things as they are when they are called to pass through trials, and to suffer what they call sacrifices, they would acknowledge them to be the greatest blessings that could be bestowed up them." (Brigham Young ,*Discourses of Brigham Young*, p. 345).

President James E. Faust during the October 1996 general conference said, "Many who think that life is unfair do not see things within the larger vision of what the Savior did for us through the Atonement and the Resurrection. Each of us has at times agony, heartbreak, and despair when we must, like Job, reach deep down inside to the bedrock of our own faith.. The depth of our belief in the Resurrection and the Atonement of the Savior will, I believe, determine the measure of courage and purpose with which we meet life's challenges."

There is someone we can always turn to, who will always be there, who will always understand.. The Savior willingly gave his life for us.

In Alma 7:11, 12

"And he shall go forth, suffering pains and afflictions and temptations of every kind; and this that the word might be fulfilled which saith he will take upon him the pains and the sicknesses of his people.

Verse 12, - - - - -"and he will take upon him their infirmities, that his bowels may be filled with mercy, according to the flesh, that he may know according to the flesh how to succor his people according to their infirmities."

Alma the Younger who suffered many trials and afflictions after his conversion testified to his son Helaman.

"I do know that whosoever shall put their trust in God shall be supported in their trials, and their troubles, and their afflictions, and shall be lifted up at the last day." (Alma 36:6)

Alma knew what he was talking about, he explains briefly some of the trials.

"And I have been supported under trials and troubles of every kind, yea, and in all manner of afflictions; yea, God has delivered me from prison, and from bonds, and from death; yea, and I do put my trust in him, and he will still deliver me." (Alma 36:27).

Because Alma is keeping the commandments and putting his trust in God, he has exceeding great faith.

"And I know that he will raise me up at the last day, to dwell with him in glory; yea, and I will praise him forever" - - - -
(Alma 36:28)
This great INNER PEACE WILL HELP US IN OUR TRIALS. Also the Lord will help ease our burdens.

As Alma and his people were in bondage to Amulon and the Lamanites , after much prayer the Lord told them in Mosiah 23

Verse 13. "And it came to pass that the voice of the Lord came to them in their afflictions, saying; Lift up your heads and be of good comfort, for I know of the covenant which ye have made unto me; and I will covenant with my people and deliver them out of bondage.

V. 14. "And I will also ease the burdens which are put upon your shoulders, that even you cannot feel them upon your backs, even while you are in bondage; and this will I do that ye may stand as witnesses for

121

me hereafter, and that you may know of a surety that I, the LORD GOD, DO VISIT MY PEOPLE IN THEIR AFFLICTIONS.

Verse 15. "And now it came to pass that the burdens which were laid upon Alma and his brethren were made light; yea, the LORD DID STRENGTHEN THEM THAT THEY COULD BEAR UP THEIR BURDENS WITH EASE, AND THEY DID SUBMIT CHEERFULLY AND WITH PATIENCE TO ALL THE WILL OF THE LORD."

The Lord may not always take away our burdens, however He will strengthen us and help us as we turn to him in prayer and supplication. Because the Nephites bore their burdens cheerfully and with patience and with great faith----

verse 16 - ----" the voice of the Lord came unto them again, saying: Be of good comfort, for on the morrow I will deliver you out of bondage."

No matter who we are, male, female, wife, mother, father, parent, or grand parent we will have trials, challenges to help us grow. If you live in the richest mansion or the humblest hut, it matters not.
"We may feel put upon by events and circumstances- - - - - -
Yet many of these things that we feel put upon by actually constitute the customized curricula needed for our personal development. - - - We can't withdraw from all of life's courses and still really stay enrolled in school!"

- - - - -"instead of complaining, we accept (more than we do) the menu of life and what is allotted to us." Elder Neal A. Maxwell, "The Holy Ghost: Glorifying Christ", *Ensign*, July 2002, pg 59,60 '

Elder Neal A. Maxwell also said, "Regarding trials, including of our faith and patience, there are no exemptions---only variations (see Mosiah 23:21). These calisthenics are designed to increase our capacity for happiness and service. Yet the faithful will not be totally immune from the events on this planet. Thus the courageous attitudes of imperiled

Shadrach, Meshach, and Abed-nego are worthy of emulation. They knew that God could rescue them. "But if not," they vowed they would still serve God anyway (see Daniel 3:16-18).Ensign, July 2002 Pg. 59, Elder Neal A. Maxwell, "The Holy Ghost: Glorifying Christ", *Ensign*, July 2002, pg 17

Can we be as courageous as these three men, serving God and not faltering even with a death sentence hanging over them. This was death by fire, one of the most painful ways to die. What courage it took to say, we will only serve the true and living God, He can save us , BUT IF NOT -- they knew, there was no doubt about their testimony.

Our challenge today, what if we are keeping all the commandments, have 100% home or visiting teaching, have scriptures and prayer daily, all of the list that keeps us in the service of the Lord. We have prayed and fasted mightily, to have this trial taken from us - - but it is still there.

Elder Dallin H. Oaks of the Quorum of the Twelve Apostles, in an article "He heals the Heavy Laden," *Ensign*, November 2006, 7-8 "Healing blessings come in many ways, each suited to our individual needs, as known to Him who loves us best. Sometimes a 'healing ' cures our illness or lifts our burden. But sometimes we are 'healed' by being given strength or understanding or patience to bear the burdens placed upon us."

Elder Kent F. Richards of the Seventy in talking in General Conference- "The Atonement Covers All Pain" *Ensign*, May 2011 page 17 gave this example footnote # 20. See Michael R. Morris, "Sherrie's Shield of Faith," Liahona and Ensign, June 1995, page 46.

"Thirteen-year-old Sherrie under went a 14-hour operation for a tumor on her spinal cord. As she regained consciousness in the intensive care unit, she said: "Daddy, Aunt Cheryl is here, . .. and . . . Grandpa Norman . . . and Grandma Brown . . . are here. And Daddy, who is that standing beside you? . . . He looks like you, only taller . . . He says he's your brother,

Jimmy." Her uncle Jimmy had died at age 13 of cystic fibrosis.

"For nearly an hour, Sherrie . . . described her visitors, all deceased family members. Exhausted she then fell asleep."

Later she told her father, "Daddy, all of the children here in the intensive care unit have angels helping them."

D. & C. 84:88, . . . "I will go before your face, I will be on your right hand and on your left, and my Spirit shall be in your hearts, and mine angles round about you, to bear you up."

In our hymn book "Hymns of the Church of Jesus Christ of Latter Day Saints" page 96

"Dearest children, holy angels   Watch your actions night and day, And they keep a faithful record   Of the good and bad you say. Cherish virtue!   Cherish Virtue!   God will bless the pure in heart."

President James E. Faust, in July 2002 *Ensign*, "A Priceless Heritage", page 5. In speaking of the Pioneers great trials said.

"I have wondered why these intrepid pioneers had to pay for their faith with such a terrible price in agony and suffering. Why were not the elements tempered to spare them from their profound agony? I believe their lives were consecrated to a higher purpose through their suffering. Their love for the Savior was burned deep in their souls and into the souls of their children and their children's children."

"In the difficult days of their journey, the members of the Martin and Willie Handcart Companies encountered some apostates from the Church who were returning from the West, going back to the East. These apostates tried to persuade some in the companies to turn back. A few did turn back. But the great majority of the pioneers went forward to a heroic achievement in this life and to eternal life in the life hereafter. Francis Webster, a member of the Martin Company, stated, "Everyone of us came through with the absolute knowledge that God lives for we became acquainted with him in our extremities."

In Moses 1:39 the Lord says, "this is my work and my glory to bring to pass the immortality and eternal life of man."

This is God's whole purpose to help us become like Him. How do we gain the attributes of God? We study his word, we keep his commandments. We strive to become like.

In Elder Groberg's book   "The Other Side of Heaven"
The Lord impresses on Elder Groberg's mind, to become patient you practice patience. ---------

In April 2002 General Conference , Mary Ellen Smoot, outgoing President of the general Relief Society said, "It does not take much living to find out that life almost never turns out the way you planned it. Adversity and affliction come to everyone. Do you know anyone who would not like to change something about themselves or their circumstances? And yet, I am sure you know many who go forward with faith. You are drawn to those people, inspired by them, and even strengthened by their examples."

President Harold B. Lee, in the book *Teachings of the Presidents of the church*, Harold B. Lee, pg. 211 said,

"Every soul that walks the earth, you and I, all of us whether rich or poor, whether good or bad, young or old-----every one of us is going to be tested and tried by storms and adversity, winds that we must defend ourselves against. And the only ones who won't fail will be those whose houses have been built upon the rock. And what's the rock? It's the rock of obedience to the principles and teachings of the gospel of Jesus Christ as the Master taught."

"So the all-important thing in life isn't what happens to you, but the important thing is how you take it.

Nephi explains when he was going the 3rd time to get the records from Laban, that he had faith, and his often quoted statement to his father, " I will go and do the things which the Lord has commanded, for I know that the Lord giveth no commandments unto the children of men, save he shall prepare a way for them that they may accomplish the thing which he commandeth them." 1 Nephi 3:7

Walking by faith, as did Nephi, "And I was led by the Spirit, not knowing beforehand the things which I should do." 1 Nephi 4:6

Nephi had no idea how he was going to obtain the plates, they had already failed twice, and nearly lost their lives. Yet he put his complete trust in the Lord. The Lord did not give Nephi a detailed list of what would happen, and what he was to do.

I'm sure that any of us would much have wanted a list,
 1. Go over the wall to Labans home.

 2. Walk over to his garden.

 3. There you will find a man drunk on the ground.

 4. It will be Laban.

 5. Smite Laban.

126

6. Put on his clothes

`7. You will meet Zoram, Laban's servant.

8. Speak to Zoram in Laban's voice an have him take you

   To the treasury.

9. Zoram will give you the brass plates.

The Lord does not show us step by step. We have to have faith.

As we listened to our prophet President Hinckley in April 2002 General Conference, he said, "We know not what lies ahead of us. We know not what the coming days will bring. We live in a world of uncertainty. For some there will be great accomplishments. For others disappointment. For some much of rejoicing and gladness, good health and gracious living. For others, perhaps, sickness and a measure of sorrow. We do not know. But one thing we do know; like the Polar Star in the heavens, regardless of what the future holds, there stands the Redeemer of the world, the Son of God, certain and sure, as the anchor of our mortal lives."

The Lord tells us to be cheerful , In D.& C. 98:1-3

1.Verily I say unto you my friends, fear not, let your hearts be comforted; yea, rejoice evermore, and in everything give thanks;

1. Waiting patiently on the Lord, for your prayers have entered into the ears of the Lord of Sabaoth, and are recorded with this seal and testament----the Lord hath sworn and decreed that they shall be granted.

3. Therefore, he giveth this promise unto you, with an immutable

covenant that they shall be fulfilled; and all things wherewith you have been afflicted shall work, together for your good, and to my name's glory, saith the Lord.

At the time this revelation was given the saints were being severely tested. The persucutions were mounting in Missouri, and just 17 days before this on the 20th of July 1833 a mob had gathered at the courthouse in Independence. They demanded the Mormons leave Missouri. They had called in the   leaders of the church in that area. They asked for 3 months to consider the request, that was denied. Then they asked for 10 days. The mob being in such a state refused and granted them 15 minutes.

When trials come upon us, how do we respond. Do we allow Satan to enter, and become angry, or do we turn to the Lord and seek for his help. By turning to the Lord we can feel peace amidst the storm.

In Helaman 5:12 Heleman is explaining to his sons Nephi and Lehi where to put their trust in times of trials and adversities.

"And now, my sons, remember, remember that it is upon the rock of our Redeemer, who is Christ, the Son of God, that ye must build your foundation; that when the devil shall send forth his mighty winds, yea, his shafts in the whirlwind, yea, when all his hail and his mighty storm shall beat upon you, it shall have no power over you to drag you down to the gulf of misery and endless wo, because of the rock upon which ye are built, which is a sure foundation, a foundation whereon if men build they cannot fall.

Our focus needs to be on the Savior, "Look unto me in every thought, doubt not fear not." D.& C.6:36

And as Alma explains in Alma:33:23,"And then may God grant unto you that your burdens may be light, through the joy of his Son.

Consider Joseph of Egypt, the many trials he suffered. Joseph had

128

11 brothers, they were jealous of him because Jacob their father favored Joseph, and gave him a coat of many colors. {Hebrew term may indicate simply a long coat with sleeves.)
Evidently he did not give the other brothers a coat.

Genesis 37:4 And when his brethren saw that their father loved him more than all his brethren, they hated him, and could not speak peaceably unto him.

Things get more intense when the Lord gave dreams to Joseph. Especially when the Sun and the moon and the stars bowed down to Joseph. " Jacob said, shall I and your mother and your brethren indeed come to bow down ourselves to thee to the earth?"
Verse 10
11. And his brethren envied him; but his father observed the saying. The brothers were also angry with Joseph because of the dreams he had.

Joseph's trials increased dramatically. He was 17 when his brothers wanted to kill him, but instead sold him to the Ishmaelites for 20 pieces of silver.

TRIALS (WHY?)

If Heavenly Father loves us more than we can even comprehend, why does He allow us to have trials. Physical pain, sickness, poverty , war, blindness, deformities. Add to that mental and emotional pain , anger , being betrayed, sadness, loneliness, fear, mental challenges. Being misunderstood.

Do you ever feel that your trials are so unfair? Or perhaps you and your family are the only ones with extreme difficulties. Have you ever sat in a church meeting and looked at all the perfect families. Look how well behaved their children are. They have a nice home, a nice car, and are active in church. I wish our family was like them. They don't have any problems or trials- - - -- - or do they. I once heard a Bishop say he was pleased when a new family moved into the ward. His thinking was   I wonder what abilities they have and perhaps what callings they could fill. He said after a few years as a Bishop his thinking changed.   Now it is, I wonder, what problems or challenges they have in their life.

President James E. Faust stated, "Many members, in drinking of the bitter cup that has come to them, wrongfully think that this cup passes by others. - - - - - -Every soul has some bitterness to swallow. (James E. Faust, *Ensign,* June 1998, *Ensign*, "A Second Birth"   Pg. 2

Why--- is often a question asked. Why me?   Why now? I have been trying to keep the commandments more now than at any other time in my life?

President Harold B. Lee said "Every soul that walks the earth, you and I, all of us----whether rich of poor, whether good or bad, young or old----every one of us is going to be tested and tried by storms of adversity, winds that we must defend ourselves against. And the only ones who won't fail will be those whose houses have been built upon the rock. And what's the rock? It's the rock of obedience to the principles and teachings of the gospel of Jesus Christ as the Master taught." (Harold B. Lee,*Teachings of Presidents of the Church* , , pg. 211)

Helaman explains to his sons Nephi and Lehi that trials will come and they will be fierce, yet if you build upon the rock of our Redeemer you will not fall.

"And now, my sons, remember, remember that it is upon the rock of our Redeemer, who is Christ, the Son of God, that ye must build your foundation; that when the devil shall send forth his mighty winds, yea, his shafts in the whirlwind, yea, when all his hail and his mighty storm shall beat upon you, it shall have NO POWER over you to drag you down to the gulf of misery and endless wo, because of the rock upon which ye are built, which is a sure foundation, a foundation whereon if men build they cannot fall." Helaman 5:12

Joseph Smith and 5 others were in Liberty Jail for 4 months. This was not like our prisons where there are 3 meals a day, warmth from the cold and a cot to sleep on. Liberty Jail was small, like a dungeon. The ceiling was so low that they could not stand up completely. They were in the jail over the long cold winter months, and there was little heat. The food was terrible

My husband served his mission in Missouri, he explains how piercing the cold is. It is so deep in it's penetration that it seems to chill even the bones. The Missouri River froze over while he was there. The humidity is high and it was so cold the air sparkled with the frozen water droplets. It was a very biting penetrating cold. Four months is a long time in these conditions. However Joseph's main concern was for the Saints and the persecution they were going through. Joseph was a prophet of God-- why did the Lord allow him to be in these circumstances? Why did these things happen to the Saints?

Elder James B. Martino of the Seventy, "All Things Work Together for Good," *Ensign*, May 2010, 101. Elder Martino said, " Our Heavenly Father, who loves us completely and perfectly, permits us to have experiences that will allow us to develop the traits and attributes we need to become more and more Christlike. Our trials come in many forms, but each will allow us to become more like the Savior as we learn to recognize the good that comes from each experience. As we understand this doctrine, we gain greater assurance of our Father's love. We may never know in this life why we face what we do, but we can feel confident that we can grow from the experience."

The Lord's answer , "KNOW THOU, MY SON, THAT ALL THESE THINGS SHALL GIVE THEE EXPERIENCE, AND SHALL BE

FOR THY GOOD." (D&C 122:7

"Elder Orson F. Whitney wrote: "No pain that we suffer, no trial that we experience is wasted. It ministers to our education, to the development of such qualities as patience, faith, fortitude, and humility. . . . It is through sorrow and suffering, toil and tribulation, that we gain the education that we come here to acquire." Orson F. Whitney, in Spencer W. Kinball's, *Faith Precedes the Miracle* (1972), 98. - - - As quoted by Elder Kent F. Richards of the Seventy, "The Atonement Covers All Pain" May Ensign 2011 pg. 15

Sometimes it is so difficult to understand the suffering, the hurts, the pain. Why??? ? ? Elder Neal A. Maxwell said, "Trying to comprehend the trials and meaning of this life without understanding Heavenly Father's marvelous encompassing plan of salvation is like trying to understand a three-act play while seeing only the second act. Fortunately, our knowledge of the Savior, Jesus Christ, and His Atonement helps us to endure our trials and to see purpose in suffering and to trust God for what we cannot comprehend." Elder Neal A. Maxwell, , "'Enduring Well", *Ensign*, April 1997, 'Enduring Well', page 7

The Lord is mindful and understands our troubles and concerns, our worries and fears, our hurts and pain whether they be mental or physical. Yet, God the great school master knows
that for us to grow and become more like him we need these learning experiences. As Elder Neal A. Maxwell said, "We are in the middle of a three act play, we were there for the first act, but we don't remember, for we agreed for a veil of forgetfulness to be placed over our minds. We cannot see the third act, yet that is the most glorious and rewarding if we have paid careful attention to the second act, the one we are living now, by keeping the commandments of God."

God wants us to realize the great blessings promised us for

remaining faithful and keeping his commandments, especially in times of great trials and tribulation. D. & C. 58:2-4

2. "For verily I say unto you, blessed is he that keepeth my commandments, whether in life or in death; and he that is faithful in tribulation, the reward of the same is greater in the kingdom of heaven."

God explains that he understands our feelings, that we can not comprehend all that he has in store for us.

3. "Ye cannot behold with your natural eyes, for the present time, the design of your God concerning those things which shall come hereafter, and the glory which shall follow after much tribulation."

After the trials come the blessings.

4. " For after much tribulation come the blessings. Wherefore the day cometh that ye shall be crowned with much glory; the hour is not yet, but is nigh at hand."

Jesus is trying to explain. He is telling us to have hope and faith in the great blessings that will come.

As we go through these trials we are being refined to help us become more Christ like. We are being strengthened for even greater responsibilities and trials. There is joy in overcoming and being strengthened. The Lord is preparing us with attributes that we will need to fight the battle against Satan, and remain strong. To be mighty warriors in these the last days.

Elder Joe J Christensen, of the Seventy says, "We all face difficulties at some time or another, and occasionally they are tough. But in every case, you probably find out later there was something the Lord was teaching you, something that is or will be of immense importance in your life." Joe J Christensen, "A Reason to Smile" *Ensign*, February 2002; pg. 58

Elder Joseph B. Wirthlin in October 2004 General Conference said, "Those who face the challenges of life often ask the question, "Why me?" he said, noting that the better question would be, "What could I learn from this experience?"

Then he said, "Though our trials are diverse, there is one thing the Lord expects of us no matter our difficulties and sorrows; He expects us to press on." Joseph B. Wirthlin , *Church News*, 9 Oct. 2004, pg 18.

The Lord knows exactly what he is doing. This is his work and his glory   Moses 1:39   He knows how far we can stretch, he knows what we need to become more like him. As we put our trust in him, he is there to lift and help us.

Alma explains this to his son Heleman, ----- "for I do know that whosoever shall put their trust in God shall be supported in their trials, and their troubles, and their afflictions, and shall be lifted up at the last day." Alma 36:

President James E. Faust said in an article in February 2006 *Ensign*, "Refined in Our Trials" page 7 -- "The Divine Shepherd has a message of hope, strength, and deliverance for all. If there were no night, we would not appreciate the day, nor could we see the stars and the vastness of the heavens. We must partake of the bitter with the sweet. There is a divine purpose in the adversities we encounter every day. They prepare, they purge, they purify, and thus they bless."

"When we pluck the roses, we find we often cannot avoid the thorns which spring from the same stem."

"Out of the refiner's fire can come a glorious deliverance . It can be

134

a noble and lasting rebirth. The price to become acquainted with God will have been paid. There can come a sacred peace. There will be a reawakening of dormant, inner resources. A comfortable cloak of righteousness will be drawn around us to protect us and to keep us warm spiritually. Self-pity will vanish as our blessings are counted."

As we study the lives of great men and women we see each had their share of trials and hardships. In the pre-existence we were told that we would come in contact with good and evil. I don't think Heavenly Father sugar coated this experience, yet we shouted for joy and were excited to come to earth. We knew it was a step we needed in order to gain physical bodies and to become like our Heavenly Parents. The faithful were given missions, or responsibilities to do on earth. Consider, Adam and Eve , Mary, the mother of Jesus, Joseph Smith, our prophet and leaders and each one of us. Many of our Latter Day Prophets have said that the youth of our day were reserved to come forth for such a time as this. This is not only for the youth of today. Consider how many times this was said, in years past if you were a youth 10, 20, or 40 or more years ago , This means YOU & I, we were sent in this day and age to be a mighty force of good.   To be a light in the world, to let our light shine. To stand for truth and righteousness. To be mighty warriors for God. To let those who are honest seekers of truth see a beacon, a light to be drawn to.

As the Savior taught the Sermon on the Mount, He said,
"Let your light so shine before men, that they may see your good works, and glorify your Father which is in heaven." Matthew 5:16

Many, many trials came because of those assignments. Consider Joseph Smith, if he had denied that he saw God the Father and Jesus , Satan wouldn't have had such a campaign against him, and he and his family may have led a life free from so many heartaches.

Abraham 3 22:23

President Joseph F. Smith in D. & C. section 138, explains the glorious vision which he received 3 October 1918. He saw those who were waiting for the advent of the Son of God into the spirit world, now the exciting thing is that President Smith explains who he saw. Not only many of the prophets , Adam, Abel, Noah, Daniel, Malachi, but the Nephite prophets, plus Mother Eve, with many of her faithful daughters. The exciting thing is YOU & I were there, Yes, we were there.

D. & C. 138:53 "The Prophet Joseph Smith, and my father, Hyrum Smith, Brigham Young, John Taylor, Wilford Woodruff, and other **CHOICE SPIRITS** WHO WERE **RESERVED** TO COME FORTH IN THE FULNESS OF TIMES TO TAKE PART IN LAYING THE FOUNDATIONS OF THE GREAT LATTER-DAY WORK" - - -

verse 55 "I observed that they were also among the noble and great ones who were chosen in the beginning to be rulers in the Church of God."

Verse 56 "Even before they were born, they, with many others, received their first lessons in the world of spirits and were prepared to *come forth in the due time of the Lord* to labor in his vineyard for the salvation of the souls of men."

President Spencer W. Kimball said: "In the world before we came here, faithful women were given certain assignments. . . . . While we do not now remember the particulars, this does not alter the glorious reality of what we once agreed to. We are accountable for those things which long ago were expected of us." (Spencer W. Kimball, "The Role of Righteous Women" *Ensign*, Nov. 1970, 102)

Trials come to everyone, no one is spared. Consider the lives of our prophets. President Spencer W. Kimball had great physical trials. The Lord knew President Kimball would become a prophet, yet because of cancer he had part of his vocal chords removed. How could he possibly speak with the raspy voice that was left. Yet, all of the church grew to love and appreciate President Kimball's voice and his counsel.

President Harold B. Lee knows what it is to lose your companion. In 1962 his beloved wife Fern Tanner Lee died. Three years later while he was on church assignment in the Pacific, his daughter Maurine, age 40, died suddenly. This was a great trial for Elder Lee. He spoke in General Conference shortly after she died.

"As I advance in years, I begin to understand in some small measure how the Master must have felt (in Gethsemane). In the loneliness of a distant hotel room 2,500 miles away, you, too, may one day cry out from the depths of your soul. . . . 'O dear God, don't let her die! I need her; her family needs her.' With all of the pleadings of this great, humble man, it was not to be. The Lord said no and took Maurine home. "God grant that you and I may learn obedience to God's will, if necessary by the things which we suffer." (Harold B. Lee, *In Conference report*, Oct. 1965, 130-131)

Enduring through these very difficult trials, elder Lee explains how they brought him closer to the Savior. "Sometimes when you are going through the most severe tests, you will be nearer to God than you have any idea." (Harold B. Lee, *Conference Report*, Munich Germany Area Conference, 1973, 114)

Trials can bring us closer to the Savior. In the Ensign, Sept.2002, One couple explains their great trial with a wayward son. "Letting Go Without Giving Up" Pg 8,10. Name Withheld. This couple were blessed with 2 children, a boy and a girl. Their daughter has remained steady and strong in the gospel, yet the son with his mental illness chose illegal drugs and substance abuse.

"Our son moved out of the house shortly after graduation from high school and began living a lifestyle totally foreign to us. We worried that he was now using drugs regularly."

"His illness was the major cause of his substance abuse and greatly complicated any recovery attempts. Our lives became a roller coaster as our son took us on a wild ride of ups and downs. ----------Every day seemed to bring a new crisis, and every phone call seemed to bring unwelcome news: "I quit my job,"   "I'm in jail," "Someone stole my paycheck,"   "My car has broken down," "I have hepatitis."   I often felt completely drained and wondered if our years of fasting and prayers were making any difference."

Discouragement set in, a feeling that nothing would help. As they read D&C 6:14 "The Spirit whispered that our son was indeed being helped by our fasts."

"At first I tried to override my son's agency with my prayers."- - - - - - - -My husband and I came to realize that we needed to learn to control our own feelings, attitudes, and reactions to his choices."

They could not have gospel discussions with their son, but they found other ways to share their testimony. They created their home to be silent sermons. On their walls are hung pictures of the Savior, and of temples , and of framed cross-stitched scriptures . Whenever the son comes home he sees the faith and testimony of his parents, without them saying a word about it.

"Living with our son's mental illness and substance abuse has not been easy, but through my experiences I have come to know and love my Savior more deeply. I have found that the only way to find true peace and happiness is by putting my trust in Him."

There is a refining process that happens when we endure our trials well. We begin to have more love for our Savior, and all of the suffering he went through for us..Our respect, love and admiration increase for this

138

wonderful older brother who gave his life that we might live. Through suffering we can become more compassionate, and understanding and less judgmental.

The dedicatory prayer that was given at the Kirtland Temple was given by revelation to the Prophet Joseph Smith. The Saints had suffered so very much at the hands of enemies. Building the temple was a huge sacrifice of both their limited finances and their physical labors and contributions.

In D.&C. 109

75. "That when the trump shall sound for the dead, we shall be caught up in the cloud to meet thee, that we may ever be with the Lord;

76. "That our garments may be pure, that we may be clothed upon with robes of righteousness, with palms in our hands, and crowns of glory upon our heads, and reap eternal joy for all our sufferings.

"*Reap Eternal joy for all our sufferings*." There are rewards, there are blessings. Sacrifice brings forth the blessings of heaven."

Chapter 8

ATTITUDE

ATTITUDE- --- BE-ATTITUDE

Have you ever said, or heard anyone say, He makes me so mad! I am so angry at that person for what they did. They make me so upset. If they would just change-- then I wouldn't be miserable any more. If my spouse would change, then I would be happy. If my children would change , then I would be happy. If my neighbor would change then I would be happy. If my neighborhood changed, then I would be happy. If the world changed to fit my expectations, - - - - - then I would be happy.

No one is changing--------stop the world I want to get off.

Pinocchio from Walt Disney's movie was a puppet and wanted to be a real live boy, finally it came true through many hard earned experiences. His actions were no longer determined by someone else pulling his strings. He sings this little song.

"I've got no string to hold me down,
   to make me fret or make me frown.
   I had strings, but now I'm free
   there are no stings on me.

HI - - O - - the ME - - RI- - - O ,
I'm as happy as can be ,
I want the world to know, nothing ever worries.
I've got no strings, so I have fun ,
I'm not tied up to anyone.
How I love my liberty, There are no strings on me."

Are you letting someone else pull your strings? Are you in reaction rather than your own action. Do you really want to give others that much control of your life?

The Savior said, "These things I have spoken unto you, that in me ye might have peace. In the world ye shall have tribulation: but be of good cheer; I have overcome the world." John 16:33

The law of Moses was an eye for an eye and a tooth for a tooth. Jesus taught the higher law. In 3 Nephi 12:21,22

"Ye have heard that it hath been said by them of old time, - - - - - -
Thou shalt not kill: and whosoever shall kill shall be in danger of
the judgement of God;

But I say unto you, That whosoever is angry with his brother
shall be in danger of his judgement."

The law of Moses was a lesser law , you were judged strictly on your actions. Jesus gave the higher law , you are judged by your thoughts. All action is proceeded by thought. The Lord is telling us to control our thinking. In the Beattitudes the Lord is telling us how to be happy. He is

141

telling us how, in spite of the trials and tests and difficulties of this life we can be of good cheer.

Harold B. Lee explains what the word Blessed means as the Savior gave in the Sermon on the Mount.

"In that matchless Sermon on the Mount, Jesus has given us eight distinct ways by which we might receive this kind of joy. Each of his declarations is begun by the word 'Blessed.' Blessedness is defined as being higher than happiness. 'Happiness comes from without and is dependent on circumstances; blessedness is an inward fountain of joy in the soul itself, which no outward circumstances can seriously affect.' () (Harold B. Lee, "Decisions for Successful Living", *Dummelow's Commentary* p. 56)

President Lee continues,
1. Blessed are the Pour in Spirit.
"To be poor in spirit is to feel yourself as spiritually needy, ever dependent upon the Lord.

2. Blessed Are They That Mourn
To mourn, as the Master's lesson here would teach, one must show that 'godly sorrow that worketh repentance' and wins for the penitent a forgiveness of sins and forbids a return to the deeds of which he mourns."

3. Blessed Are the Meek
A meek man is defined as one who is not easily provoked or irritated and forbearing under injury or annoyance. Meekness is not synonymous with weakness. The meek man is the strong, the mighty, the man of complete self-mastery. He is the one who has the courage of his moral convictions, despite the pressure of the gang or the club."

4. Blessed Are They That Hunger and Thirst After Righteousness
"Did you ever hunger for food or thirst for water when just a

crust of stale bread or a sip of tepid water to ease the pangs that distressed you seem to be the most prized of all possessions? If you have so hungered then you may begin to understand how the Master meant we should hunger and thirst after righteousness."

5. Blessed Are the Pure in Heart

"You can see only that which you have eyes to see. Some of the associates of Jesus saw him only as a son of Joseph the carpenter. Others thought him to be a wine-bibber or a drunkard because of his words. Still others thought he was possessed of devils. Only the righteous saw him as the Son of God. Only if you are the pure in heart will you see God, and also in a lesser degree will you be able to see the 'God' or good in man and love him because of the goodness you see in him.

6. Blessed Are the Merciful

"Our salvation rests upon the mercy we show to others. Unkind and cruel words, or wanton acts of cruelty toward man or beast, even though in seeming retaliation, disqualify the perpetrator in his claims for mercy when he has need of mercy in the day of judgment before earthly or heavenly tribunals. Is there one who has never been wounded by the slander of another whom he thought to be his friend? Do you remember the struggle you had to refrain from retribution? Blessed are all you who are merciful for you shall obtain mercy!"

7. Blessed Are the Peacemakers

"Peacemakers shall be called the children of God. The troublemaker, the striker against law and order, the leader of the mob, the law-breaker are prompted by motives of evil and unless they desist will be known as the children of Satan rather than God.--------That one who is quarrelsome or contentious, and whose arguments are for other purposes than to resolve the truth, is violating a fundamental principle laid down by the Master as an essential in the building of a full rich life. 'Peace and good will to men on earth' was the angel song that heralded the birth of the Prince of Peace."

8. Blessed Are They Which Are Persecuted

"May youth everywhere remember that warning when you are hissed and scoffed because you refuse to compromise your standards of abstinence, honesty and morality in order to win the applause of the crowd. If you stand firmly for the right despite the jeers of the crowd or even physical violence, you shall be crowned with the blessedness of eternal joy. Who knows but that again in our day some of the saints or even apostles, as in former days, may be required to give their lives in defense of the truth? If that time should come, God grant they would not fail!"

(Harold B. Lee, *Decisions for Successful Living*. pp 56-63)   I found this information in the church study guide, "The Life and Teachings of Jesus and His Apostles) pages 60 & 61

In verses 43-46 of 3rd Nephi, chapter 12 the Savior talks about our human response to those who hurt us.

"And behold it is written also, that thou shalt love thy neighbor and hate thine enemy; But behold I say unto you, love your enemies, bless them   that curse you, do good to them that hate you, and pray for them who despitefully use you and persecute you;"

The Savior is teaching us or rather commanding us to control our mind. He is telling us that we can choose our response. He acknowledges that this person (enemy) has cursed you. They do hate you. That they have actually despitefully used you and persecuted you. These are some very painful things that the enemy has or is doing to you.

The Savior's response to what is happening to us, He knows it is unfair, and not right. He doesn't say to get revenge, or angry, or hate them. He gives us four action words. LOVE -- - BLESS - -DO GOOD - - - PRAY - - -. Now who are these words for, for us to use. Our first response

144

would be; of course, I can do that to my friends, and those who love me and are kind to me. That would be easy, and you are probably already doing that.

But wait, Jesus said to "Love your enemies" How????The human part of us wants to get revenge, to get even, to hurt them the way we have been hurt. The Lord show's us how to change our thinking, or focus, our thoughts. We can learn to love them by BLESSING THEM , by DOING GOOD to them, by PRAYING FOR THEM.

How does this help. First of all are we keeping the commandments? As we do this we will be blessed with His Spirit and inner peace. We change our focus from negative to positive. We are blessed because we do not allow bitterness and anger in our hearts. We are not consumed with revenge. As we strive to have more love, we will feel more of the Lord's Spirit. We focus on helping rather than hurting. We ask the Lord to help us let go of the hurt and pain and to fill our lives with love.. We choose to forgive, help, and lift others.

A modern day example of loving your enemies and praying for those who despitefully use you and persecute you is a true story taken from the "New Era," October 1994, pages 44 & 45. The article is entitled "Pray for Her" by Richard M. Romney.

Ava Rosenberg was 12 years old. She enjoyed her friends and school. One day she was surprised when another girl her age tried to pick a fight over a pen that she said Ava had taken from her. Of course Ava would never do such a thing and told her she must be mistaken for she did not take the pen. Things might have been O.K. but they escalated when the girl's older sister got involved. This older sister was involved with a gang and had a long criminal record. These two sisters were from a home where the father was an alcoholic, and the mother often was not there. They were on their own much of the time. They did not have the love and guidance

145

and support of loving parents.

The older sister threatened to harm Ava. She made threats like "You had better watch out and keep your back side covered, You took my sister's pen, and I'm going to get you for doing that." "I know what your class schedule is and I will be waiting for the opportunity to teach you a lesson."

She was concerned that they might attack her, so she asked to stay in the classroom during lunch. Ava was always on the lookout for these sisters, and was as careful as possible to not be alone. Several weeks later when Ava left the classroom to get a drink of water she saw them, she could see by the look on their faces that they were angry and meant her harm. There was no where to run or get protection. They grabbed her, then kicked her in the stomach, and punched her jaw. It happened so fast Ava had no defense. The pain was intense as she struggled to breath from being kicked in the stomach- then they punched her in the jaw. Ava could not believe they were treating her this way. Their anger was so intense almost a rage against her. As if this was not enough for the sisters, They grabbed her and continually beat her head into the ground.

There was much pain and many unsuccessful operations, and finally they put a titanium plate in her jaw. Ava had been released from the hospital on a Saturday, the next day was fast and testimony meeting. Ava went to church and even though it was difficult for her to speak she went to the pulpit.

"The scars from my injuries will heal," Ava said. "But the girl who attacked me has deeper scars inside. I have a loving family and the gospel to get me through. She has neither. Pray for her . Pray that the missionaries can find her and teach her, so that she can turn from hate to love."

"We're supposed to love our enemies," she says matter-of-factly. "When I was in the hospital, I couldn't speak because I was in so much pain. But I could think, and I remember thinking to myself. What would the Savior do?"

Three years after the attack she say's, "I will probably have a plate in my jaw all my life. But it doesn't matter because I know I will be healed in the celestial kingdom. I just hope and pray that my assailant will be healed too."

The Lord gave us the gift of moral agency. We choose what we think about. We may not always be able to choose what happens to us. Ava, certainly did not choose to be beaten up. She certainly did not choose to be hurt and in so much pain., but her first thoughts in the hospital were, "What would the Savior do." She patterned her life after our perfect example, Jesus Christ. She prayed for her enemy and asked others to add their prayers also..We have the freedom to cho0se our response. Ava chose to focus on the blessings she has now, her loving family , the gospel and knowing her body would be healed, that she would not forever be in pain with a metal plate in her jaw. It is our response - - - - our response-ability. To chose carefully our thoughts.
Because Ava chose to forgive and pray for her enemy she was lifted from a burden, a heavy mental load

God will take the trials, and difficulties and heartaches, and help us learn from them. To become stronger and better people. This story explains how a trial can actually be a great blessing.

THE BUTTERFLY

"A man found a cocoon of a butterfly. He took it home So that he could watch the butterfly come out of the Cocoon. One day a small opening appeared. He sat and watched the butterfly for several hours as the butter-fly struggled to force its body through that little hole. Then it seemed to stop making any progress. It appeared as if it had gotten as far as it could and it could go no further. It just seemed to be stuck. Then the

147

man, in his kindness, decided to assist the butterfly so he took a pair of scissors and snipped off the remaining bit of the cocoon. The butterfly then emerged easily. But it had a swollen body and small, shriveled wings. The man continued to watch the butterfly because he expected that, at any moment, the wings would enlarge and expand to be able to support the body, which would contract in time. Neither happened! In fact, the little butterfly spent the rest of its life crawling around with a swollen body and shriveled wings. It never was able to fly. What the man, in his kindness, did not know was that the restricting cocoon and the struggle required for the butterfly to get through the tiny opening were God's way of forcing fluid from the cocoon. Freedom and flight would only come after the struggle. By depriving the butterfly of a struggle, he deprived the butterfly of health.

Sometimes struggles are exactly what we need in our life. If God allowed us to go through our life without any obstacles, He would cripple us. We would not be as strong as we could have been

We all must endure trial, and hardships, heartaches and disappointments. The all important thing in life isn't what happens to you, but the important thing is how you take it and what you learn from it!!"
Author unknown

Some people go around being miserable. You comment on the weather , it is either too hot or cold, or sunny or rainy for them. If you ask them how they feel- look out they may tell you, every ache and pain even to explaining in detail their last 10 operations. Also they remember and will tell you if you will listen, what Johnny did to them 16 years ago, when they were in school. How someone slighted them , they did not get promoted for a job that they deserved. There parents always loved one of their siblings more then them. How unfair life is. It seems like something miserable happens to them every day.

When Jesus walked the earth there was much oppression from the

Roman Government, and also from the Jewish leaders, He knows that soon he will leave earth life and He knows the trials that his apostles and disciples will have. In John 16:33 he says,

"These things I have spoken unto you, that in me ye might have peace. In the world ye shall have tribulation: but be of good cheer; I have overcome the world."

In the D.&C. 61:36, "And now, verily I say unto you, and what I say unto one I say unto all, be of good cheer, little children; for I am in your midst, and I have not forsaken you;" The Lord is telling us what attitude to have, and the reason we can have a good attitude is because Jesus is in our midst. In the Savior is where we find, joy and peace and help.

President Hinckley our beloved prophet has the responsibility and the weight of a world wide church. I'm sure there must be many pressures and decisions, but President Hinckley keeps focused on the Lord.

"It isn't as bad as you sometimes think it is. It all works out.
Don't worry." I say that to myself every morning. " It will all work out. If you do your best, it will all work out. Put your trust in God and move forward with faith and confidence in the future. The Lord will not forsake us. He will not forsake us,. . . . If we will put our trust in Him, if we will pray to Him, if we will live worthy of His blessings, He will hear our prayers." { President Gordon B. Hinckley, From the priesthood session, Jordan, Utah South Regional Conference, March 1, 1997}
President Hinckley understands that each one of us has trials, and doubts and fears. He gives this counsel.

"I have little doubt that many of us are troubled with fears concerning ourselves. We are in a period of stress across the world. There are occasionally hard days for each of us. Do not despair. Do not give up. Look for the sunlight through the clouds. Opportunities will eventually

149

open to you. Do not let the prophet of gloom endanger your possibilities."
(Ensign April 1986, 4-5}

D. & C. 78:17, 18
"Verily, verily, I say unto you, ye are little children, and ye have
not as yet understood how great blessings the Father hath in his own hands
and prepared for you;

"And Ye cannot bear all things now; nevertheless, be of good cheer,
for I will lead you along. The kingdom is yours and the blessings thereof
are yours, and the riches of eternity are yours."

Our attitude is so important. How we look at things. Do we allow
our mind to dwell on positive or negative things.

The Lord in D.& C. 98:1 says, "Verily I say unto you my friends,
fear not, let your hearts be comforted; yea, rejoice evermore, and in
everything give thanks;"

This is not a suggestion, this is a commandment. We are to realize
that there is a purpose for all of our learning experiences.

Continuing on in D.& C. 98, the Lord says in verse 3
". . . . .and all things wherewith you have been afflicted shall work
together for your good, and to my name's glory, saith the Lord."

President Hinckley says, " I am asking that we stop seeking out the
storms and enjoy more fully the sunlight. I am suggesting that as we go
through life we "accentuate the positive." I am asking that we look a little
deeper for the good, ...

"What I am suggesting is that each of us turn from the negativism
that so permeates our society and look for the remarkable good among
those with whom we associate, that we speak of one another's virtues

more than we speak of one another's faults, that optimism replace pessimism, that our faith exceed our fears." (President Hinckley, *Ensign*, April 1986, 2-4}

The Lord explains this in D. & C. 136:28, 29   The Saints are camped at Winter Quarters by the Missouri River, near Council Bluffs, Iowa.. It is January 1847, and it is cold, extremely bone chilling, below freezing weather. The saints don't have their, R.V.'s with a heater inside, plenty of food picked up at the local grocery store, and lots of warm weather clothing. They have been robbed by their enemies , they were driven out of their homes to flee as best they could. The situation was serious and life threatening.   The Lord was completely aware of their plight, and how difficult it was for them. Yet he did not wave a magical wand, and suddenly they were in Salt Lake with beautiful homes. He knew the growth that would come from these experiences, he did not take away their learning opportunity. In His kindness and love he told them how to do their best in their trying times.

Verse 28. " If thou art merry, praise the Lord with singing, with music, with dancing , and with a prayer of praise and thanksgiving.

29. "If thou art sorrowful, call on the Lord thy God with supplication, that your souls my be joyful.

As the pioneers traveled toward their promised land in the Rocky Mountains they endured many hardships. A covered wagon, is very small, perhaps the size of a large S.U. V. The pioneers did not have nearly the material possessions that we have today. Yet there were basic necessities in order to survive. Food, bedding, plow, seeds, etc.

Prophets of old have looked forward to our day, when the gospel would be restored in it's fullness. We are here to help prepare a people ready to receive their Savior. Satan's powers have been unleashed. The forces are gathering. We are on the Lord's side. Let us rejoice in this great

151

work the Lord wants us to do. He wants us to BE OF GOOD CHEER AND DO NOT FEAR! (D. & C. 68:6)

ATTITUDE

I woke up early today, excited over all I get to do
before the clock strikes midnight.

I have responsibilities to fulfill today, I am important.
My job is to choose what kind of day I am going to have.

Today I can complain because the weather is rainy, or - - - -
I can be thankful that the desert is getting watered.

Today I can feel sad that I don't have more money or - - - -
I can be glad that my finances encourage me to plan my
purchases wisely and guide me away from waste.

Today I can grumble about my health or - - - - - -
I can rejoice that I am alive.

Today I can lament over all that my parents didn't give me when I
was growing up, or - - - -
I can feel grateful that they allowed me to be born.
Today I can cry because roses have thorns, or - - -
I can celebrate that thorns have roses.

Today I can mourn my lack of friends or - - - -
I can excitedly embark upon a quest to
discover new relationships.

Today I can whine because I have to go to work, or - - -

I can shout for joy because I have a job to do.

Today I can murmur dejectedly because I have to do
house work, or - - -
I can feel honored   because God has provided shelter
for my mind, body, and soul.

What today will be like is up to me.
I get to choose what kind of day I will have.

HAVE A GREAT DAY .....
UNLESS YOU HAVE OTHER PLANS.

Author unknown.

God has given us the ability to think, we have the freedom to
choose what ever thought we want. As was said before we may not be able
to choose what happens to us but we can chose how we will respond.

"Nothing bad happens in a persons life without an equal or greater
benefit coming in return. Pain will do only one of 2 things, either it will
push us to the furthest point from our dreams, or it will draw us closer to
them than any other circumstance could.. The choice is ours."   (Art E.
Berg, Finding *Peace in Troubled Waters*,)

Elder Marion D. Hanks, an emeritus member of the First Quorum
of the seventy: gave this example in the Ensign, Nov. 1990 pg. 38,
"Changing Channels"

"A father is aboard an airplane on a a short business trip. He has
with him his five-year-old son and is almost wishing his son were not
there because it is a very rough trip. There are downdrafts and updrafts
and head winds alternating with tail winds, and some passengers are
feeling a bit queasy. Apprehensively, the father glances at his son and
finds him grinning from ear to ear.

"Dad, he says, "do they do this just to make it fun for the kids?"

The story is told of a young man, Tom who moved to a new area. This was many years ago, and the towns were not very large. As Tom was approaching the village he saw an elder gentleman sitting by the entrance. Here was his opportunity to ask him what the people were like since this man had probably lived there some time. "Sir, would you please tell me about the people here, what are they like, is this a good place to reside in?"

The man studied Tom a few minutes, raised his brow, and said, " young man would you describe for me what the people were like in your home village.?'

This seemed like a very unusual question for Tom , what difference did it make? Why would the old man even care about his previous home. As Tom thought about it, his eyes got dark, and a scowl slid on his face.

"Why, you can't imagine how awful it was. The villagers were mean, and unkind. They would talk about you behind your back. If you weren't careful they would even steal your sheep, or things from your home. You had to be on guard every minute. They would lie about you and gossip, I don't think there was one nice person there. I'm so glad I don't live there any more.

The old man pondered, then looked Tom in the eye. "Well young man, I'm afraid this village won't be what you wish. You will find those who steal, lie, are unkind and some are just downright mean. It will be a lot like the place you just described."

Tom's shoulders slumped as he slowly walked away.
Several days later we find the grey haired man again sitting by the entrance . Since he knew everyone in the area, when he saw a middle aged man approaching he knew he was new to these parts.

154

John was tall, and had a pleasant look on his face, even though he was tired form the day's travel. He reached out his hand to the elderly man, and introduced himself. "Sir, you seem as though you might have lived her sometime. Would you give me your ideas on what I can expect from this community? Is this a good place to live? You see I want a pleasant area for my wife and children."

The aged man studied him carefully, and said, "Well John, would you tell me what the villagers were like where you used to live?"

John's eyes brightened, there was a cheerfulness in his voice. "Why, yes sir, I would be glad to. You see, it was the most pleasant village you could imagine. Everyone was kind, why if you needed extra help with your crops, someone was always volunteering, almost with out you even asking. You see this was small hamlet was not a wealthy area, but everyone seemed to have enough and to spare. One really dry season our crops didn't do well, and we didn't have a lot to eat. Almost as if by magic, someone would bring over extra turnips, or greens, potatoes, and even milk from their own cow.

The old man smiled and said, "Why that is just like this valley! I think you will love it here!".

So much of our thinking is habit. Some people start the day with , I hate my job , I don't want to go to work. The boss is mean the customers dis-satisfied. What a lousy day. I'd quit my job but I have all these bills to pay.   (This person is focusing on the negative)

Recognize what you are think about, pay attention to it.

President James E. Faust, as he quotes from "The Secret Garden" by Frances Hodgson Burnett

The Lord wants us to be happy, in fact Elder Joe J. Christensen (of the Seventy) say's,

"We should remember that happiness is a commandment and not merely a suggestion." *Ensign*, February, 2002 p. 58 "A Reason to Smile."

There are many scriptures where the Lord has commanded us to be happy. D.& C. 61: 36

"And now, verily I say unto you, and what I say unto one I say unto all, be of good cheer, little children; for I am in your midst, and I have not forsaken you; " D. & C. 68:6, wherefore, be of good cheer, and do not fear, for I the Lord am with you, and will stand by you; - - - - - - -"

We all have trials and challenges to face, how can we still be happy, or have inner peace. Victor Frankl, in his book , 'Man's Search for Meaning,' who lived in concentration camps said, "We who lived in concentration camps can remember the men who walked through the huts comforting others, giving away their last piece of bread. They may have been few in number, but they offer sufficient proof that everything can be taken from a man but one thing: the last of the human freedoms---to choose one's attitude in any given set of circumstances.

Glenn Van Ekeren from his book "The Speakers Source book , pg. 60 , added this - - -

"You and I can also be liberated by unlocking the resources of our mind. Dr. Frankl lived the belief that life is 10 percent what happens to us and 90 percent how we respond to it. You choose!"

A Professor at B.Y.U. was talking about attitude, and how it affects us, our mental and emotional state. He gave a few examples of what happened in his life, then one of his students gave this example. I'll call the girl Stephany. Stephany was planning on shopping at her favorite store, she had some much needed items to pick up. This was a very popular business and finding a parking space was sometimes a challenge She hoped there would be fewer customers that day but the parking lot was full, not one empty space Stephany drove slowly around the lot confident that soon someone would leave and she could quickly pull in. The minutes ticked by as she slowly drove and looked. It was so frustrating in not finding anything.

Finally after 15 minutes she saw an empty space, the only problem she was on the other side and would have to drive all the way around. She knew that was her spot, because of all the driving and waiting she had done. It almost had her name on it to reserve it for her. She hurriedly drove to the other side and just as she was almost there, another car took her space. "How could anyone do that! This is not fair! I'm going to give them a piece of my mind. I'm so angry, they did this just for spite. They knew I was heading to get this parking spot. How thoughtless and rude they are."

She screeched on her brakes just behind the offender , threw the car door open, and marched right up to the culprit. Just then the driver turned around , and Stephenie screamed - - "Aunt Suzie, this was her favorite Aunt.

President Spencer W. Kimball stated, "Happiness does not come by pressing a button, as does the electric light; happiness is a state of mind and comes from within. It must be earned. It cannot be purchased with money; it cannot be taken for nothing."
Spencer W. Kimball, *Ensign*, October 2002, "Oneness in Marriage" pg. 40

President James E. Faust, said, "You can have great meaning and purpose in your lives, even in the profane world in which we live. You can have strength of character so that you can act for yourselves and not be acted upon." (See 2 Nephi 2:26) (President James E. Faust, *Ensign*, July 2002, 'A Priceless Heritage', pg. 6)

The Lord has given us a formula for being happy. In D.& C. Section 98
Attitude is so important. How do we keep the proper attitude with so many challenges. This life is real and the challenges are real. By putting our trust in Heavenly Father and our Savior Jesus Christ. We can't comprehend the great blessings that are in store for us.

The Savior tells us in D.& C. 78:17,18

"Verily, verily, I say unto you, ye are little children, and ye have not as yet understood how great blessings the Father hath in his own hands and prepared for you;

18. And ye cannot bear all things now; nevertheless, be of good cheer, for I will lead you along. The kingdom is yours and the blessings thereof are yours, and the riches of eternity are yours.

Also in D.& C 79:4 "Wherefore, let your heart be glad- -- - ---- - - and fear not, saith your Lord, even Jesus Christ. Amen."

Attitude is so very important. How we look at things. Roses are beautiful, one of God's creations, the rose bud opens to reveal a colorful blossom, that has such a sweet fragrance. The colors are as the hues in a rainbow. Yet is the rose without fault. Have you ever counted the thorns on one single stem, or pricked your finger. Each rose may have up to ten thorns, yet what do we focus on, the beauty and fragrance of the blossom. As we inhale the sweet aroma, and gently touch the velvet pedals, we hear a voice from the rose. You are wrong to admire me, the pedals are not the real me, look I have faults. Each thorn represents one of my imperfections, there is dust on my blossoms , I have a sharp tongue, when you pick me, I will prick you with my sharp thorns which will hurt you. Once you pick me, I will only last a week or two, my blossoms will wilt but the thorns will still be there. I cannot enjoy the compliments or accept them, you see I am focused on my thorns. Now I begin to see only the thorns, I no longer see the beauty.

There are some people who think it is wrong to accept a compliment, or to take joy in who they are, and the talents God has given them. They feel it is being prideful, or not humble. Think of a time you admired a talent or quality, or ability in someone, or the way they dressed, the outfit they have on. Mary, that is a beautiful dress. You look very nice in it. Mary's reply, "Oh this old thing. I have had it for years, and look you can see a tiny flaw here. The color is not right for me." You were giving Mary a gift, and this gift seemed to be thrown back in your face. You even feel a little embarrassed that you brought it up. You now don't feel happy, and neither does Mary.

Can you graciously accept a compliment? Thank you and a smile is all that is needed. If you really feel you don't deserve the compliment, then mentally take the time to think wow I really appreciated what they said. I still don't think I deserve the compliment, but I will continue to make progress in that area. They admired something about me, I will take this gift and treasure it.

President James E. Faust said, "In Roselandia Brazil, outside the great city of Sao Paulo, there are many acres of beautiful roses. When one stands on a small hill above the rose fields, the aroma is delightful and the beauty is exhilarating. The thorns on the bushes are there, but they in no way lesson the enjoyment of the sight and the smell. I would challenge all to put the thorns, slivers, and thistles we encounter in life in proper perspective. We should deal with them but then concentrate on the flowers of life, not on the thorns. We should savor the smell and beauty of the flowers of the rose and the cactus. To savor the sweet aroma of the blossoms, we need to live righteous and disciplined lives in which the study of the scriptures, prayer, right priorities and right attitudes are integrated into our lives. (James E. Faust,"To Receive a Crown of Glory", *Ensign*, pg. 6)`

Our lives are like the rose, we each have beauty, talents and abilities. No one is perfect, no one can do everything perfectly. Yet we need to take these talents and let them shine., as in the scripture, " let your light so shine before men, that they may see your good works, and glorify your Father which is in heaven." Matthew 5:16

Think of your talents, what are your gifts? Magnify you talents. The most common ones that come to mind are, sports, music, arts, crafts, but there are many others, you don't have to be in the lime light to have a talent. Patience, being a good listener, compassion, faith, organization, kind, loving, supportive, generous. In D. & C. 46 many gifts are listed, and in verse 26 And all these gifts come from GOD FOR THE BENEFIT OF THE CHILDREN OF GOD.

Have an Attitude of Gratitude. God has commanded us to be thankful, it is not just a suggestion, but a commandment. Have you even done something nice for someone perhaps sent a gift for a wedding or birthday, or you took the time to make the quilt, or the cookies or whatever, you knew they would like. You smile as you wrap the gift, knowing they will be very pleased. Even though you can not be there you know they will be excited to receive what you gave. Several weeks pass, you know they have received your gift. You begin to question, did they really like it - you wonder. You never receive a thank you. You had joy in giving the gift, but now you feel short changed.

One of the joyful, yet sad things recorded in the scriptures is when Jesus healed the ten Lepers. In the days of Jesus being a leper was being an outcast. To understand more we look in the Bible Dictionary, page 723 & 724

" Leprosy is a terrible form of skin disease, still common in dry climates, and highly contagious.. Lepers were forbidden by the law to enter any walled city. If a stranger approached, the leper was obliged to cry "unclean." The disease was regarded as a living death, and indicated by

160

bare head, rent clothes, and covered lips."

The flesh on their hands & faces and entire body was being eaten away with this dreaded disease. This disease could cause paralysis, ulceration, gangrene, and mutilation. With their physical bodies deformed, They were outcast, that is why they stood afar off. It was the law, to protect others. They lived on their own, in groups of people who had this painful, slow, way to die. They could no longer be with their families, the mental and physical suffering they had to endure. They knew there was no hope, all was gone except the certainty of death. If they met someone they had to say , unclean - or in other words, don't get near me. They were looked down upon.

These lepers heard of the miracles of Jesus, they began to have hope, could he heal them, would he heal them? Would they find Him? In one of the villages they saw Jesus walking on the road.

In Luke 17:11-18 it is recorded "And it came to pass, as he went to Jerusalem, that he passed through the midst of Samaria and Galilee.

"And as he entered into a certain village, there met him ten men that were lepers, which stood afar off: When they heard of the miracles that Jesus had done, they had a glimmer of hope. When they saw Him they still had to keep their distance, they yelled - because they were not legally to get near Him. "And they lifted up their voices, and said, Jesus, Master, have mercy on us. "And when he saw them, he said unto them, Go shew yourselves unto the priest. And it came to pass, that as they went, they were cleansed. Can you imagine the joy and the excitement they saw and felt.

They began to feel different, their skin was becoming whole, clean and fresh. Smiles were on their faces as they saw and felt the difference for themselves and each other. To be able to mingle with the people, to again be with their families, to no longer be condemned, or have to shout unclean. Nine of them hurried to show themselves to the priests. Not even thinking to thank the giver of the gift, freedom from Leprosy, the disgrace, the humiliation.

As the lepers were going as quickly as possible to show themselves to the Priest, Jesus saw one of them turn back , he was so grateful. "And one of them, when he saw that he was healed, turned back, and with a loud voice glorified God, "And fell down on his face at his feet, giving him thanks: and he was a Samaritan. And Jesus answering said, Were there not ten cleansed? But where are the nine?

"There are not found that returned to give glory to God, save this stranger. How sad that the things these lepers wanted most, to be able live and be cured, they took no thought to thank the one who gave them the miracle. God does notice and wants us to give thanks. He wants us to tell Him , He wants us to be grateful. Being thankful puts us in a positive frame of mind. We are more happy, and life is more joyful.

There are even more blessings for us if we keep a thankful heart . In D. & C. 78:19 "And he who receiveth all things with thankfulness shall be made glorious; and the things of this earth shall be added unto him, even an hundred fold, yea, more."

President Monson, "The Divine Gift of Gratitude"   November 2010 *Ensign* , October Conference 2010, Often we feel grateful and intend to express our thanks but forget to do so or just don't get around to it."

President Monson quoted   a statement from William Arthur Ward, in Allen Klein, comp., Change Your Life! (2010), 15. Someone has said that "feeling gratitude and not expressing it is like wrapping a present and not giving it."

There is the story of a man, who just lost his wife. She was a wonderful woman, someone commented to him that he must have told her a lot of his love for her. "Nope, he said, I told her when I married her that I

162

loved her, and that was enough, and if I ever changed my mind I would let her know. How late is too late. When someone dies suddenly at times we wish we had said more to let them know of our appreciation and love for them

John Kralik from his article "Thank You!" Guidepost May 2011, pages 14, 16,17

He starts out by saying, "SOME PEOPLE WAKE UP happy. I'm not one of them." John explains why he is miserable, he was on his second divorce, and his girlfriend had just walked out on him, plus his apartment was so small that he was embarrassed to have his 7 year old daughter come and visit him. He hardly ever visited with his two grown sons, and his law firm he had started was doing terrible. John was going to go hiking with his girlfriend that day, but now she was gone. He decided to go anyway.

It was New Years Day, and everyone was watching the Rose Parade, but all John wanted to do was get away from marching bands, and the sounds. Finally, peace and quiet, but he took a wrong turn, he was lost. It seemed to fit, he figured he had lost his way in life also , he needed to figure this out. He was miserable, why? "Then I heard a voice, a loud, clear voice, saying, "Until you learn to be grateful for the things you have, you will not receive the things you want." Who was talking to me? There was no one around."

John thought about his grandfather, who gave him a gift of a silver dollar, John was 5 at the time. Now his grandfather was very wise, he said "I will give you another, if you send me a letter thanking me for this one." Even at the young age of 5 John realized this was a pretty good deal, so he sent the thank you letter, and soon received another silver dollar. But soon the thank you's were forgotten and the silver dollars stopped. As John was trying to find the right trail, ideas came into him mind, why had the silver dollars stopped, was that because he no longer

163

thanked the giver of the gift. He decided on a plan, this was the beginning of a new year, maybe he could write a thank you note every day for this new year.

A good place to start was the Christmas gifts, he wanted to thank his son, and was ready to address the letter, but realized he didn't even have his address, he had not even been to his apartment. So calling his son, they reconnected and planned on lunch together. John has been writing expressions of appreciation for two years, and has now written over 700 thank you notes. If he finds himself getting depressed or having negative thinking he can immediately change his thoughts to positive by looking at over 700 blessings he has received.

Ideas - - Song Count Your Blessings, pg. 241
Article, Thank You *GuidePosts* May 2011 pg. 14

Our attitude affects everything we do. What we have learned, how we view the world, how we analyze or process each situation. Our attitude is shaped by what we have experienced, the positive and negative things that have happened in our life, from infancy to the present day. It can be just a comment from a someone we meet for a minute, but usually it is from an authority figure, or someone we believe are all knowing. Parents have the wonderful opportunity of directing and shaping their child, with love, direction, guidelines, positive input, experiences to help them grow and develop into productive, caring adults who contribute their talents and abilities to help their families and others. Teachers fall into this category , as do siblings, friends, school mates etc. But unfortunately there are many who don't.

"You will never learn - - You are so stupid ---- How could you - - You can't sing, it is best if you just mouth the words. Etc. So our mind set is I can't do it, I will never succeed, I will not sing I can't   - - -

Jane (not real name)   Is a leader in an organization, where her skills are good and needed. She sits up front with the other leaders, she looks unhappy, sad. It is hard to figure out if she is mad at someone, or if she just stubbed her toe and is in a lot of pain. Her expression is sadness, she rarely smiles. Meeting her on the street, or in the store, it is the same and she explains the challenges she or others she feels responsible for are having. How she is angry with this person or frustrated with another, or how difficult this situation is. You walk away feeling wow she has a lot of challenges, no wonder she never smiles.

Jane explained an experience she had recently, she was in the temple, going over in her mind her concerns, worries , trying to figure out solutions. After the session a lady came over to her and said , "You seem so sad , I just wanted you to know God loves you and will help you."

(My thought was, what a caring woman to notice Jane and come up and give words of encouragement.) I was amazed at what Jane said next. "Can you believe that woman, she thought I was sad and depressed. I don't appreciate her telling me to not be sad. I feel that people that go around with a smile on their face are FAKE , they are not real , they are just putting a pasted smile on. They are not living in the real world." Wow , that answered my question, Jane's attitude, her value system is you are counterfeit. if you have a happy, joyous attitude and countenance.

Everyone, and that is everyone has challenges, difficult decisions, hardships, etc, but lets look to our current day prophets. President Hinckley, and President Monson. They had or have the responsibilities of being President of the Church of Jesus Christ of Latter Day Saints, that includes all it's members, and to warn, invite, encourage, the whole world.

In General Conference Oct. 2011, one of the General Authorities, or Seventy, told of being weighed down with his new calling, how could he possibly fulfill his responsibilities. He was very discouraged , he got on the elevator of the church office building and was just staring at the floor, someone got on , and saw his gaze at the bottom of the elevator. He said,

165

"What are you looking at?" " Oh nothing was his response."   Then he looked up and saw the Prophet. President Monson said with a big smile on his face, "I find if you look up it will help."

Chapter 9

ATONEMENT

Whatever Jesus lays HIS HANDS UPON LIVES. IF JESUS
LAYS HIS HANDS UPON A MARRIAGE, IT LIVES. IF HE IS
ALLOWED TO LAY HIS HANDS ON THE FAMILY, IT LIVES."
President Howard W. Hunter , General Conference, 1979
(Church News-----29 December 2001)

The most loving act of kindness, The Atonement was given us by
the Father and His Son. Our Savior Jesus Christ. The plan of Happiness
from the beginning involved the fall. "For as in Adam all die, even so in
Christ shall all be made alive." 1 Corinthians 15:22

Abinadi explains beautifully the Atonement in Mosiah. Abinadi's
very life was at stake, wicked King Noah and his priest would have killed
him before he delivered his message, but because of the power of the Lord
they could not even touch him at that time.

God would not allow Abinadi to be smitten until he had delivered
this wondrous message of the Atonement. Only one person of all the
wicked priests of Noah was converted;   Alma! How the Lord's work was
furthered because of this message being delivered.

"Touch me not, for God shall smite you if ye lay your hands upon
me, for I have not delivered the message which the Lord sent me to
deliver." - - - - - - Mosiah 13:3

V. 6   "And he spake with power and authority from God: - -

Abinadi , then quotes from Isaiah 53:3-5 which is written in Mosiah   14: 3-5, "He is despised and rejected of men; a man of sorrows, and acquainted with grief; and we hid as it were our faces from him; he was despised, and we esteemed him not.

"Surely he has borne our griefs, and carried our sorrows; yet we did esteem him stricken, smitten of God and afflicted. But he was wounded for our transgressions, he was bruised for out iniquities; the chastisement of our peace was upon him; and with his stripes we are healed."

In verses 10-12, it further explains how much Jesus paid for us; he gave everything.

"Yet it pleased the Lord to bruise him; he hath put him to grief; when thou shalt make *his soul an offering for sin* -- - - -

"He shall see the travail of his soul; and shall be satisfied; by his knowledge shall my righteous servant justify many; for he shall bear their iniquities.

"Therefore will I divide him a portion with the great, and he shall divide the spoil with the strong; because *he hath poured out his soul unto death*; he was numbered with the transgressors; and he bore the sins of many, and made intercession for the transgressors."

The last supper, the eve before Jesus was crucified, He knew what was in store for him, Yet He tells his disciples "In the world ye shall have tribulation: but be of good cheer, I have overcome the world." John 16:33

Knowing the pain, the suffering, all the things that were to come upon him, that he would carry everyone's sins, hurts, sorrows, injustices, how could he possible say, be of good cheer. Perhaps it is a tiny bit like when a woman knows her time is near and she is about to go into labor,

168

she knows there is intense agony that is soon coming and will keep getting more poignant, for hours at a time, till finally a baby is born. Then she rejoices, for a new child of God is brought into the world.

Elder Neal A. Maxwell, expounds on this telling the many things that would impact on the Savior. "The unimaginable agony of Gethsemane was about to descend upon Jesus; Judas' betrayal was imminent. Then would come Jesus' arrest and arraignment; the scattering of the Twelve like sheep; the awful scourging of the Savior; the unjust trial; the mob's shrill cry for Barabbas instead of Jesus; and then the awful crucifixion on Calvary. What was there to be cheerful about? Just what Jesus said: He had overcome the world! The atonement was about to be a reality. The resurrection of all mankind was assured. Death was to be done away with---Satan had failed to stop the atonement." (Neal A. Maxwell, *But a Few Days* (1983), 4.

Our Heavenly Father provided a way for us to learn and grow and in order to become like him we needed to obtain a physical body. Coming to earth gave us our bodies, now we need to learn to control our physical bodies. To have our spirit body take control over our physical appetites. To learn and recognize the good from the evil and choose the good.

Sheri L. Dew explains, "The Lord knows the way because He *is* the way and is our only chance for successfully negotiating mortality. His Atonement makes available all of the power, peace, light, and strength that we need to deal with life's challenges--those ranging from our own mistakes and sins to trials over which we have no control but we still feel pain." (Sheri L. Dew, "Our Only Chance"'*Ensign*, May, 1999, pg 67 '

God knew we would make mistakes on our earthy journey, so a plan was provided so we could learn and grow. But since no unclean thing can enter the Kingdom of God, and we have all made mistakes how could we ever return to be in His presence again.

169

The Bible Dictionary page 617 has a wonderful explanation of the Atonement. "Atonement. The word describes the setting "at one" of those who have been estranged, and denotes the reconciliation of man to God. Sin is the cause of the estrangement, and therefore the purpose of atonement is to correct or over come the consequences of sin."
Elder Adhemar Damiani said, "Atoning means suffering the punishment for sin, thus removing the effects of the transgression of the repentant sinner and allowing him or her to be reconciled with God. Jesus Christ was the only one capable of making a perfect atonement for all humankind." Elder Adhemar Damiani, , "The Merciful Plan of the Great Creator" pg. 11, *Ensign*, March 2004
There is a story from "The Speaker's Source book" by Glenn Van Ekeren, pg. 312,313.

TWICE MINE

"Oh, he was proud. The little boy held up his boat and declared, "It's all mine. I made every part of you." Then he made his way to the shore of the lake. This was the day he had been waiting for. His handmade masterpiece skipped along the clear, blue water as the gentle breeze caught the sails. Suddenly, a gust of wind caught the boat and snapped the string the little boy was holding. It was out of control and beyond the boy's reach, until finally it disappeared in the middle of the lake. Heartbroken, the little boy made his way home---without his prized sailboat. It was gone!

Several weeks later, the little boy was walking down Main Street. As he passed the toy shop, something caught his eye. There it was! How could it be? There in the window was his toy boat. He rushed into the store and told the owner the story of his boat. "It really is mine," he said. "I made it with my own two hands." The shopkeeper shook his head and said, "I am sorry. That is my boat now. If you want it back, you'll have to pay the price."

Dejected, yet hopeful, the boy left the toy shop, determined to buy back his boat. He worked and saved doing any job that friends, neighbors, and family would provide.

Finally, the day came. His heart danced as he entered the toy shop and spread his hard-earned money on the counter. "I want to buy my boat back," the boy said. The owner carefully counted all the change and a few dollar bills. There was enough. Reaching into the showcase window, the store owner carefully retrieved the little boat and placed it in the boy's outstretched hands.

The little boy walked into the afternoon sun and hugged his boat. "You're mine," he said. "Twice mine. First I made you, and then I bought you."

Why are we important? Because first God made us, and then He bought us. "

Elder Jeffrey R. Holland, member of the Quorum of the Twelve Apostles, said in General Conference April 2002, "I testify that no one of us is less treasured or cherished of God than another. I testify that He loves each of us- - - insecurities, anxieties, self-image, and all. He doesn't measure our professions or our possessions. He cheers on every runner, calling out that the race is against sin, not against each other.. I know that if we will be faithful, there is a perfectly tailored robe of righteousness ready and waiting for everyone, "robes . . . . . made . . . white in the blood of the Lamb."

"Christ's Atonement , of course, is for super sinners and the midrange sinners and then good people who make a lot of mistakes but are not wicked."   Elder Neal A. Maxwell, "The Holy Ghost: Glorifying Christ." July 2002, *Ensign* p.56

Sheri L. Dew gave insight into the Atonement. "Our responsibility is to learn to draw upon the power of the Atonement. Otherwise we walk through mortality relying solely on our own strength. And to do that is to invite the frustration of failure and to refuse the most resplendent gift in time or eternity."- - - - - - - - - - -

Elder Tad R. Callister (of the Seventy) Dec. 2010 *Ensign*, Article - - "Fear Not"

"Because of the Savior's birth, life, and Atonement, there are no unsolvable problems. There are temporary tragedies and difficulties, of course, but they need not be permanent or unconquerable. Can you imagine anyone having a problem God cannot solve? He always has a solution that will advance our eternal progress. That is both the reason for and essence of the Atonement." "if you believe in the Atonement and do God's will, you need not fear because there will always be a solution to your problems."

"Negativism and cynicism stem from Satan. Cheerfulness and optimism stem from Christ."

Elder Callister explains that all of our problems fit into four categories.

"First, **death** - -"For as in Adam all die, even so in Christ shall all be made alive."
(1 Corinthians 15:22).

Second, **sin**. - - - Jesus would "save his people from their sins" (Matthew 1:21).

Third, **weakness**. The Savior taught Moroni that His "Grace (the enabling power of the Atonement is sufficient for all men that humble themselves before me; for if they Humble themselves before me, and have faith in me, then will I make weak things become strong unto them" (Ether 12:27).

172

Fourth, **common ailments of life that may be unrelated to sin** (such as sickness, Rejection, depression, loss of employment, and so forth). Isaiah prophesied that The Savior would "bind up the brokenhearted," "comfort all that mourn," and "Give unto them beauty for ashes" (Isiah 61:1-3; see also Alma 7:9-13).

"For every affliction the world throws at us, the Savior has a remedy of superior healing power."

Christ did not have to suffer. There was no law that bond him. He did not have to pay the price of sin - - BECAUSE HE WAS SINLESS. I do not like pain of any kind, either physical or mental or emotional. It is not pleasant, it is so uncomfortable, it is PAINFUL. Why would Christ suffer for me? Why would he willingly suffer for my sins, not only for me, but for everyone who has or will live on this earth. This must amount to billions of people. Yet this is not all, he took upon himself the suffering of all of God's creations , worlds without number. Why? Because of His great love for us.

Alma explains this in the Book of Mormon, Alma 7:11,12.

"And he shall go forth, suffering pains, and afflictions and temptations of every kind; and this that the word might be fulfilled which saith he will take upon him the pains and the sicknesses of his people. - - - - and he will take upon him their infirmities, that his bowels may be filled with mercy, according to the flesh, that he may know according to the flesh how to succor his people according to their infirmities."

King Benjamin in his speech to the Nephites who were gathered near the temple explains in more detail the sufferings of the Savior, for you and for me.

Mosiah 3:7   "And lo, he shall suffer temptations, and pain of body, hunger, thirst, and fatigue, even more that man can suffer, except it be

unto death; for behold, blood cometh from every pore, so great shall be his anguish for the wickedness and the abominations of his people."
Jesus rarely says anything about the pain and suffering he went through, but we get a small insight when we read in D. &C. 19:16-19

16. "For behold, I, God, have suffered these things for all, that they might not suffer if they would repent;

17. "But if they would not repent they must suffer even as I;

18. "Which suffering caused myself, even god, the greatest of all, to tremble because of pain, and to bleed at every pore, and to suffer both body and spirit----and would that I might not drink the bitter cup, and shrink----

19. "Nevertheless, glory be to the Father, and I partook and finished my preparations unto the children of men."

None of us can imagine, can comprehend the agony or tremendous sufferings, physical, mental, and emotional.

In the footnotes of May 2011 page 17 number 13 Elder Kent F. Richards of the Seventy in the article "The Atonement Covers All Pain" In this article Elder Richards said "Christ *chose* to experience pains and afflictions in order to understand us."
He also quotes from President Henry B. Eyring "Adversity," *Liahona and Ensign*, May 2009, 24: emphasis added. President Henry B. Eyring taught: "It will comfort us when we must wait in distress for the Saviors's promised relief, that He knows, from experience, how to heal and help us . . . .And faith in that power will give us patience as we pray and work and wait for help. **He could have known how to succor us simply by revelation, but He chose to learn by His own personal experience."**

174

13. See John Taylor, The Mediation and Atonement (1882), 97, President Taylor writes of a "Covenant" being entered into between the Father and the Son in the premortal councils for the accomplishment of the atoning redemption of mankind. Christ's voluntary suffering during life was in addition to the suffering in the garden and on the cross (see Mosiah 3:5-8) "Likewise, the Lord is our advocate, and He "knoweth the weakness of man and how to succor them who are tempted."(D&C 62:1 In other words, He knows how to succor all of us. But we activate the power of the Atonement in our lives. We do this by first believing in Him, by repenting, by obeying His commandments, by partaking of sacred ordinances and keeping covenants, and by seeking after Him in fasting and prayer, in the scriptures, and in the temple." President Taylor,"Our only Chance". *Ensign*, May 1999, pg 67

Elder Richard G. Scott of the Quorum of the Twelve Apostles said, "I've realized that, though my life isn't fair at times, I can cast my cares on the Savior. The Atonement will not only help us overcome our transgressions and mistakes, but in His time, it will resolve all inequities of life----those things that are unfair which are the consequences of circumstance or others' acts and not our own decisions."(Elder Richard G. Scott "Jesus Christ, Our Redeemer," *Ensign*, May 1997, p54).

Elder Joseph B. Wirthlin in General Conference October 2004, said   I know there are many who suffer heartbreak, loneliness, pain, and setback. These experiences are a necessary part of the human experience. However, please do not lose hope in the Savior, and His love for you. It is constant and He promised that He would not leave us comfortless." Joseph B. Wirthlin, *Church News*, 9 Oct. 2004, pg 18

Because of the Savior's Atonement , our sins, hurts, pains injustices, tears, can all be healed. We can have joy, now in this life even with our trials, and pain. Consider Moroni, he had no family, no friends for about 22 years , yet he focused on the Lord and added great things to the Book of Mormon to help us. Moroni wanted to share with us, his faith , hope, belief in our Savior Jesus Christ.

Elder Richard G. Scott in his Conference address, "The Atonement can Secure Your Peace and Happiness" *Ensign*, Nov. 2006 , Pg. 41 & 42 says, "Each of us makes mistakes in life. They result in broken eternal laws. Justice is that part of Father in Heaven's plan of happiness that maintains order. - - - - - It is a friend if eternal laws are observed. - - - - - Justice guarantees that you will receive the blessings you earn for obeying the laws of God. Justice also requires that every broken law be satisfied. When you obey the laws of God, you are blessed, but there is no additional credit earned that can be saved to satisfy the laws that you break. If not resolved, broken laws can cause your life to be miserable and would keep you from returning to God. Only the life, teachings, and particularly the Atonement of Jesus Christ can release you from this otherwise impossible predicament."

"The demands of justice for broken law can be satisfied through mercy, earned by your continual repentance and obedience to the laws of God. Such repentance and obedience are absolutely essential for the Atonement to work its complete miracle in your life.

The Redeemer can settle your individual account with justice and grant forgiveness through the merciful path of your repentance. Through the Atonement you can live in a world where justice assures that you will retain what you earn by obedience. Through His mercy you can resolve the consequences of broken laws."

Made in the USA
Columbia, SC
08 September 2019